DR. ATKINS'
NEW
CARBOHYDRATE
GRAM COUNTER

DR. ATKINS' *NEW* CARBOHYDRATE GRAM COUNTER

ROBERT C. ATKINS, M.D.

More than 1,300 brand-name and generic foods listed with total carbohydrates, fiber, Net Carbohydrates,* protein and fat content, plus calories

**The only carbs you need to count when you do Atkins*

M. Evans and Company, Inc.
New York

M. Evans and Company, Inc.
216 East 49th Street
New York, New York 10017

Library of Congress Catalog Card Number : 96-61523

Design and type formatting by Bernard Schleifer

Printed in the United States of America

15

Contents

Foreword

Why Publish a New Edition?

In the six years since this book was first published, more and more people have embraced the idea of limiting carbohydrate intake for weight control—as well as overall good health. Numerous scientific studies have corroborated the logic of the Atkins philosophy. Meanwhile, as the twin epidemics of obesity and diabetes have picked up pace, mainstream health professionals are increasingly realizing that achieving a healthy weight is not just a matter of cutting back on fat and calories. There is a growing awareness that sugar, white flour, trans fats and the junk foods made with them are a large part of the problem.

To make this book more useful, we've made a host of improvements:

- **Use of a new software program.** This system enables us to provide more precise nutritional information.
- **More data.** We provide not just grams of carbohydrate, but also Net Carbs. These are the only carbs you need to count when you do Atkins because they exclude carbohydrates such as fiber and sugar alcohol, which have a minimal impact on blood sugar. Although there is no need to count calories if you are counting

carbs, many people find it psychologically gratifying to know how many calories they are consuming so we have added them as well.

• **More controlled carb foods.** Bagels made with soy flour and pancake mixes made with wheat gluten and starch-resistant maize contain a fraction of the carbs found in white flour versions. Comparable offerings among breakfast cereals, breads, muffins, crackers and even pasta allow you to enjoy such traditional foods without overloading on sugar and starch.

• **Other new products.** We also have added or increased our inclusion of soy products, pastas made from grains other than wheat and brands such as Newman's Own and Far East that now are commonly found on grocery shelves.

• **More vegetables.** This section has been considerably amplified, acknowledging the importance of these most nutrient-dense carbohydrates, so you can select those lowest in carbs.

• **More categories.** To make it easier for you to find what you are looking for, we've divided previous grouped food categories such as "Desserts and Snacks" into two. Within categories, we've made entries more logical. Now, for example, pork loin and ham appear under a pork heading, instead of scattered alphabetically throughout an overall meat listing.

• **New sections.** These short chapters help with the practicalities of eating out. "Dining Out" allows you to make informed choices among a wide variety of ethnic cuisines. "Fast Foods" offers assistance in navigating the treacherous waters—carbwise—in such establishments. You'll learn how to estimate portions when you are not in your own kitchen in "Portion Size Guidelines."

This revised edition of *Dr. Atkins' New Carbohydrate Carb Counter* is the perfect companion to the recently revised best-selling *Dr. Atkins' New Diet Revolution*, which reflects Dr. Atkins' latest thinking and current terminology. The changes are not just linguistic. The name of Atkins Nutritional Approach™ (instead of the Atkins diet) reflects the fact that eating controlled carbohydrate foods is actually a prescription for a permanent healthy lifestyle. Seven new chapters clarify the Atkins approach, with twice as many references as the former edition, 100 brand new recipes and tips for making it easier than ever to follow the program. You may also want to read *Dr. Atkins Quick & Easy Cookbook*, written with Veronica Atkins. For more information on these books and the Atkins Nutritional Approach™, go to *www.atkinscenter.com*.

Introduction

Congratulations! If you've purchased this book, you've made a decision to pursue the controlled carbohydrate path to weight control. But you may not yet realize that you will likely also enjoy improved energy and better health by following the Atkins Nutritional Approach™.

We know you can't wait to get started. If you are already limiting your carbohydrate intake, you already understand that it's a proven way to once and for all take control of your weight. But Atkins is much more. *Dr. Atkins' New Diet Revolution* fully explains the four principles upon which it is based. But in brief, by doing Atkins for a lifetime, you can:

• **Lose weight.** Achieving optimal weight is an important component of good health.

• **Maintain that weight loss.** The problem with most diets is not that they don't work, but that they don't last. When doing Atkins, you gradually add back carb foods until you reach the level of carbohydrate intake that allows you to maintain a healthy weight.

• **Achieve good health.** When doing Atkins, nutritional needs are met with wholesome, whole foods.

• **Lay the groundwork for disease prevention.** Controlling carbs lowers insulin levels, which lowers risk factors for chronic diseases, including heart disease, hypertension, diabetes and certain cancers.

Understanding these principles makes it clear that Atkins is not just a diet that you start when you have a few pounds to lose and stop when you reach your goal. Four phases (described on pages 15–16) enable you to gradually change your eating habits, resulting in a lifetime of slimness. Doing Atkins also allows you to establish an eating program that is individually tailored to your needs, based on your age, gender, metabolism and level of physical activity.

Carbohydrates Versus Calories and Fat

The reason that millions of copies of *New Diet Revolution* have been sold and that millions of individuals swear by Atkins is very simple: It works. Even if you've failed on low-fat diets, once you understand that the real culprit is an over-reliance on carbohydrate foods, particularly those full of sugar, refined flour and other processed ingredients, you are on the path to success. In the last two decades, three things have happened:

• Our culture has been obsessed with dietary fat.
• Low-fat and fat-free products proliferated—many of them junk foods loaded with white flour, sugar and other nutrient-deficient ingredients.
• Nonetheless, by eating these foods Americans have become fatter than ever.

The culprit is not fat per se; it's the over-consumption of carbohydrates. Obviously, counting calories and restricting fat intake has not worked. The average individual now consumes upwards of 300 grams of carbs a day, far too much for most people to metabolize (burn as energy). When you eat foods high in carbs, your body converts them to glucose, or blood sugar, which is released into your blood stream. Your pancreas then releases the hormone insulin, which transports the glucose to your cells. Whatever is not used for energy is stored as fat.

When blood glucose levels become elevated, the pancreas responds with a flood of insulin. Keep this up for years and your body can become incapable of utilizing the insulin efficiently. This metabolic disorder, called insulin resistance or hyperinsulimia, can be a precursor to diabetes. Being overweight, particularly very overweight, raises the risk of developing this condition. Insulin is known as the fat-producing hormone so excess insulin can lead to excessive fat. Fortunately, the solution to excessive insulin production is simple: Control carbohydrate intake.

A Metabolic Switch

The Atkins approach is fundamentally different than the low-fat approach to weight loss. Both carbohydrate and fat provide fuel for the body's energy needs. If carbohydrate is available, the body burns it as fuel first, but burning fat is also perfectly natural and safe. Switch your body from a glucose metabolism to a mostly fat metabolism, and you burn your body fat for energy instead of storing it. It is crucial that you understand that it's not simply *dietary* fat that makes you fat. Rather, it's excess carbohydrates, especially in the form of sugar, white flour and other starches—found in breads, pasta, and potatoes and in almost all over-processed convenience foods and snacks.

Where Carbs Lurk

When you do Atkins, eating proteins, healthy fats and nutrient-dense carbohydrates helps stabilize your blood sugar so you don't get ravenously hungry or depleted of energy a few hours after eating. Most of us are unfamiliar with the sources of carbohydrates and their relative merits. In fact, many people think that only grains and sweets are carbohydrate foods and don't realize that they are found in milk, fruits and even vegetables. That's why this *Carbohydrate Gram Counter* is of immediate help in two important ways.

First, success in doing Atkins is dependent upon accurately calculating the carbohydrate grams consumed each day. To do this with ease, you need a handy reference guide so that your decisions are based on facts, not assumptions. Secondly, although manufactured foods carry a Nutrition Facts Panel mandated by the Food and Drug Administration, it can still be difficult to ascertain the actual Net Carbohydrate gram count of each food. The panel lists total grams of carbohydrates as well as the grams of dietary fibber. Subtract the dietary fiber from the total and you will have a rough idea of the Net Carbs, although this figure does not usually factor in sugar alcohol and definitely not glycerine, which have minimal impact on blood sugar. Moreover, if a label lists 0 g of carbohydrate, it can actually be as high as 0.99 g. It is also important to check the serving size upon which the calculations are based. You may find that a single serving is considerably smaller than the portion you are actually eating. Still, the Nutritional Panel information is a valuable adjunct to this carb gram counter and it is worth getting in the habit of reading food labels. They are a great way to become aware of the staggering amount of sugar in many foods. In the near future, these labels are expected to include trans fats broken out from the total fat. At this time, the only way to ascertain if trans fats are in a food is to search the list of ingredients for hydrogenated fat or partially hydrogenated fat.

It's important that you understand that we have included foods in the *Carbohydrate Gram Counter* that are not recommended on the Atkins Nutritional Approach™ so you can compare them with foods more appropriate to doing Atkins. Please also understand that a book of this size cannot be comprehensive. Although it is impossible to list every product or every flavor of each product, we have provided enough basic information so that (in concert with Nutritional Panel information), you can guesstimate the carb counts for specific items not listed herein.

Let me leave you with three more pieces of important advice. Be sure to drink at least eight 8-ounce glasses of water a day to flush out your system and avoid dehydration or constipation. No matter what eating plan you choose to follow, a good multi-vitamin/mineral supplement ensures you get the recommended daily intake of all nutrients. And to complement and speed your weight loss, be sure to get plenty of exercise.

My *Carbohydrate Gram Counter* will make it easier than ever to do Atkins and I have every confidence that the changes in this edition will make it even more useful and user friendly.

—ROBERT C. ATKINS, M.D.

A Brief Look at the Four Phases of the Atkins Nutritional Approach™

1. Induction: This initial phase, the most restrictive of carbohydrates, jump-starts weight loss. You eat no more than 20 grams of Net Carbs per day, which translates into roughly 3 cups of salad greens and other non-starchy veggies. You can eat liberal amount of protein (meats, fish, poultry, eggs) and healthy fats. Atkins is not a license to gorge. When you're hungry, eat the amount that makes you feel satisfied but not stuffed. Stay on Induction for a minimum of two weeks.

2. Ongoing Weight Loss: When you move to OWL, you deliberately slow your weight loss as you introduce more variety in nutrient-dense carbohydrate foods. So long as weight loss continues, you gradually increase your carb intake in the following manner: Week one, eat 25 grams of carbs per day; week two, move to 30 grams of carbs per day, and so forth, until weight loss stalls. Then back down to the previous level. This threshold is known as your Critical Carbohydrate Level for Losing (CCLL).

Choose your additional carbs wisely, first from vegetables low in carbohydrates, then from other fresh, healthful, nutrient- and fiber-rich sources. Typical 5-gram increments include 10 Brazil nuts, half an avocado or 1/2 cup of green beans. Then add berries, which are lower in carbs than other fruits. Some individuals can add back legumes and whole grains, as well as other fruits. Typical daily tolerance levels range anywhere from 30 to 90 grams of carbohydrate. The more you exercise, the more carbs you can handle.

3. Pre-Maintenance: When your weight goal is in sight, you move to this phase and increase your daily carb allotment in 10 gram increments each week until weight loss slows to one or two pounds a month. This excessively slow pace is deliberate as you internalize eating habits that become part of a permanent lifestyle for weight maintenance.

4. Lifetime Maintenance: When you reach your goal weight, you are officially in this phase. Depending upon your age, gender, activity level and genetics, you can likely consume anywhere from 90 to 120 grams—or even more—of carbs per day. This threshold is your Critical Carbohydrate Level for Maintenance (CCLM). Most people can occasionally eat modest portions of foods such as potatoes and other starchy vegetables, and regular (not controlled carb) whole-wheat pasta and wholegrain bread without regaining weight. On the other hand, extremely metabolically resistant individuals may never be able to go beyond, say, 30 grams of carbs. No matter what your CCLM, for good health, continue to avoid white flour, sugar and all junk foods.

These four phases are fully described in *Dr. Atkins' New Diet Revolution*, along with lists of acceptable foods and suggested menus for each phase.

How to Use This Book

We made this book pocket-sized for a very good reason. It should travel with you to the grocery store, your place of work, to the finest restaurants and—without question—to fast food places. At home it will help you plan meals. Making up menus and a shopping list before you head off to the supermarket will keep you on track. Stick to your list and you will not be tempted by foods that don't belong in your meals—and in your house. You will find you can simply avoid certain grocery aisles full of carb-filled foods. This book may be small, but the import of its content is huge. Refer to it regularly and you will begin to understand how little things add up and how seemingly small changes can make a significant difference.

If you've been on low-fat diets, you've undoubtedly counted calories. You may have also counted grams of fat. With Atkins, you count grams of carbohydrate, a job made easy with this handy guide. Although we have provided information on fat, protein and calories for reference, the main thing you need to concern yourself with is a food's Net Carb count. These are the only carbs that count when you do Atkins. Unlike total carbs, they don't include the fiber, sugar alcohols and glycerine that have little impact your blood sugar levels. (Also keep an eye on fiber content to ensure that your have adequate roughage in your diet. Fiber also slows the entry of glucose into your blood stream, reducing blood sugar spikes and helps rid your body of cholesterol.)

Build your meals around protein foods such as meat, fish, poultry and eggs, vegetables and healthy fats such as olive oil and other monounsaturated fats. There is no need to restrict fat so long as you are controlling your carb intake. The one exception is trans fats, the hydrogenated oils found in most margarines and many packaged foods. Butter is a much healthier option. Check labels for trans fat and pass up anything that contains it. Your body is unable to process this unnatural fat.

Plan your daily or weekly menus by picking foods with low carbohydrate counts. But this is not just a numbers game. Twenty grams of carbs from a jelly doughnut do not equal 20 grams from three cups of salad and other vegetables. Always select fresh, natural foods instead of refined, over-processed ones. Avoid anything made with white flour and sugar—and that includes most junk foods. When counting carbs, be sure to include those in snacks, beverages and artificial sweeteners.

The advice in this book is not meant to be a substitute for the advice of your personal physician. If you are embarking on a weight-loss program, you should see your doctor first.

CAUTION: The advice offered in this book, although based on the author's experience with many thousands of patients, is not intended to be a substitute for the advice and counsel of your personal physician. If you are currently taking diuretics, insulin or oral diabetes medications, consult your physician before starting Atkins. You will need to reduce and then closely monitor your dosage as you lower your blood-sugar level. People with severe kidney disease should not do Atkins. The weight loss phases of the Atkins Nutritional Approach are not appropriate for pregnant women and nursing mothers.

Portion Size Guidelines

Even on Atkins, it's important to be able to judge portion size, especially for higher carb foods. How much is a half a cup? What does a three-inch slice look like? To help you recognize portions at a glance, we've created the following charts.

Bread, Grains, and Pasta

1 one-ounce slice of bread	An index card
1 two-ounce piece of Italian bread	A bar of soap
1 three-ounce bagel	1 can of tuna
¹/₂ cup rice, cereal or pasta	¹/₂ baseball
1 two-ounce muffin	A cupcake wrapper

Fruits and Veggies

1 medium fruit or ³/₄ cup cut-up fruit	A tennis ball
1 cup green salad	A fist
¹/₂ cup cooked vegetables	A scoop of ice cream

Protein and Cheese

2 tablespoons peanut butter	Two tea bags
3 ounces beef, chicken or pork	A small pack of tissues or cigarettes
1 ounce of cheese	A pair of dice
1 ounce of nuts	Two ping pong balls or a small child's handful

Snacks and Desserts

1 ounce of chips	A medium-sized handful
1 three-inch piece of cake	A small stack of business cards
1 cup of ice cream	A baseball

Measurements

1 tablespoon	1 teabag
1 teaspoon	1 thimble
1 cup	1 fist or 1 baseball
¼ cup	1 large egg

Food Categories

BEVERAGES

Water is the most healthful beverage, but iced herbal teas and lemonades or limeades sweetened with a sugar substitute are suitable options for a change of pace. When you crave the flavor of fruit juice, purchase unsweetened concentrate (cranberry or passion fruit are good choices) in a health food store and mix with sugar substitute and water or seltzer. Some vegetable juices are a better bet: Tomato juice has only 4 Net Carbs per half-cup and contains lycopene, an important antioxidant. Remember, when you are on the Lifetime Maintenance phase and decide to splurge on a Frappucino from Starbucks, you should think of it as a liquid dessert.

Though most alcoholic drinks—with the exception of sugar-laden fruit concoctions or drinks mixed with soda—are relatively low in carbs, they should be consumed in moderation. The body burns alcohol as a fuel before fat, so drinking alcohol slows down the fat-burning process. That said, after the Induction phase, an occasional glass of wine with dinner or a light beer is an acceptable part of a controlled carbohydrate lifestyle.

Food Item (Amount)	Carb (g)	Fiber (g)	Net Carbs (g)	Protein (g)	Fat (g)	Cals
Nonalcoholic Beverages						
ATKINS SHAKE, READY TO DRINK						
Chocolate (11 oz)	5.0	3.0	2.0	20	9.0	170
Strawberry (11 oz)	4.0	2.0	2.0	20	9.0	170
Vanilla (11 oz)	4.0	2.0	2.0	20	9.0	170
ATKINS SHAKE MIX, POWDER						
Cappuccino (2 scoops)	2.0	0.0	2.0	24.0	8.0	170
Chocolate (2 scoops)	3.0	2.0	1.0	24.0	9.0	180
Strawberry (2 scoops)	1.0	0.0	1.0	24.0	8.0	170
Vanilla (2 scoops)	1.0	0.0	1.0	24.0	8.0	170
CHOCOLATE DRINKS						
Hot cocoa, Carnation, with marshmallows (1 pkt)	23.0	0.8	22.2	1.0	3.0	120
Hot cocoa, Nestle, no sugar added (1 pkt)	8.4	0.8	7.6	4.3	0.4	55
Hot cocoa, Nestle Rich Chocolate (1 pkt)	24.2	0.7	23.6	1.3	1.1	112
Hot cocoa, sugar-free, Atkins (1 pkt)	3.0	0.0	3.0	1.0	2.5	50
Nesquik Chocolate Drink (8 fl oz)	33.0	1.0	32.0	7.0	8.0	230
YooHoo (8 fl oz)	29.0	0.0	29.0	2.0	1.0	130
COFFEE (see also "Starbucks")						
Brewed (regular, decaf) (8 fl oz)	1.0	0.0	1.0	0.2	0.0	5
Cappuccino, Sugar Free Ultra Creamy Mix (3 tbs)	3.0	0.0	3.0	1.0	2.0	50
Instant powder (1 tsp)	0.7	0.0	0.7	0.2	0.0	4
GATORADE, most flavors (8 fl oz)	15.2	0.0	15.2	0.0	0.0	60

Food Item (Amount)	Carb (g)	Fiber (g)	Net Carbs (g)	Protein (g)	Fat (g)	Cals
JUICES, FRUIT						
Apple (4 fl oz)	14.5	0.1	14.4	0.1	0.1	58
Apricot nectar (4 fl oz)	18.1	0.8	17.3	0.5	0.1	70
Cranberry juice cocktail, frozen, concentrate (2 tbs)	18.6	0.0	18.6	0.0	0.0	73
Cranberry juice cocktail, light, Ocean Spray (4 fl oz)	5.6	0.0	5.6	0.0	0.0	23
Cranberry juice cocktail (4 fl oz)	18.2	0.1	18.1	0.0	0.1	72
Fruit punch (4 fl oz)	14.8	0.1	14.6	0.0	0.0	58
Grape (4 fl oz)	18.9	0.1	18.8	0.7	0.1	77
Grapefruit, sweetened (4 fl oz)	13.9	0.1	13.8	0.7	0.1	58
Grapefruit, unsweetened (4 fl oz)	11.1	0.1	11.0	0.6	0.1	47
Guava nectar (4 fl oz)	19.0	1.0	18.0	0.2	0.1	74
Lemon (2 tbs)	2.6	0.1	2.5	0.1	0.0	8
Lime (2 tbs)	2.8	0.1	2.7	0.1	0.0	8
Mango nectar (4 fl oz)	18.9	0.9	18.0	0.3	0.1	73
Orange, fresh (4 fl oz)	12.9	0.3	12.7	0.9	0.3	56
Orange, from concentrate (4 fl oz)	13.4	0.3	13.2	0.9	0.1	56
Orange Peach Mango, Dole (4 fl oz)	14.0	0.0	14.0	0.5	0.0	60
Orange Strawberry Banana, Dole (4 fl oz)	14.0	0.0	14.0	0.5	0.0	60
Passion fruit (4 fl oz)	17.8	0.2	17.6	0.8	0.2	74
Peach nectar (4 fl oz)	17.3	0.8	16.6	0.3	0.0	67
Pear nectar (4 fl oz)	19.7	0.8	19.0	0.1	0.0	75
Pineapple (4 fl oz)	17.2	0.3	17.0	0.4	0.1	70

Food Item (Amount)	Carb (g)	Fiber (g)	Net Carbs (g)	Protein (g)	Fat (g)	Cals
Prune (4 fl oz)	22.3	1.3	21.1	0.8	0.0	91
Tangerine Orange, Tropicana (4 fl oz)	12.5	0.0	12.5	1.0	0.0	55
JUICES, VEGETABLE						
Carrot (4 fl oz)	5.8	0.0	5.8	0.7	0.2	25
Clam & tomato (4 fl oz)	13.2	0.2	13.0	0.7	0.2	58
Tomato (4 fl oz)	5.1	1.0	4.2	0.9	0.1	21
Vegetable juice cocktail (4 fl oz)	5.5	1.0	4.5	0.8	0.1	23
LEMONADE						
Crystal Light, prepared (8 fl oz)	0.0	0.0	0.0	0.0	0.0	5
Prepared from concentrate (8 fl oz)	25.9	0.0	25.9	0.3	0.1	99
Prepared from powder (8 fl oz)	26.9	0.0	26.9	0.0	0.0	103
MILK, FLAVORED						
Chocolate, Reduced Fat, Hershey's (4 fl oz)	15.0	0.0	15.0	4.0	2.5	100
Double Chocolate, Nesquik (8 fl oz)	30.0	1.0	29.0	8.0	9.0	230
Strawberry, Lowfat, Parmalat (8 fl oz)	25.0	0.0	25.0	7.0	3.0	150
NANTUCKET NECTAR						
100% Apple Juice (8 fl oz)	25.0	1.0	24.0	0.0	0.0	100
Squeezed Blueberry Tea (8 fl oz)	19.0	0.0	19.0	0.0	0.0	80
Squeezed Diet Lemon Tea (8 fl oz)	0.0	0.0	0.0	0.0	0.0	0
SNAPPLE						
Cranberry Raspberry drink, diet (8 fl oz)	2.0	0.0	2.0	0.0	0.0	10

Food Item (Amount)	Carb (g)	Fiber (g)	Net Carbs (g)	Protein (g)	Fat (g)	Cals
Kiwi Strawberry juice drink (8 fl oz)	28.0	0.0	28.0	0.0	0.0	110
Tea, lemon, sweetened (8 fl oz)	22.6	0.0	22.6	0.0	0.0	88
Tea, lemon, diet (8 fl oz)	8.4	0.0	8.4	0.0	0.0	21
SODAS						
Cola (12 fl oz)	38.7	0.0	38.7	0.0	0.0	153
Diet (12 fl oz)	0.0	0.0	0.0	0.0	0.0	0
Ginger ale (12 fl oz)	31.8	0.0	31.8	0.0	0.0	124
Grape (12 fl oz)	41.7	0.0	41.7	0.0	0.0	160
Lemon-lime (12 fl oz)	38.3	0.0	38.3	0.0	0.0	147
Root beer (12 fl oz)	39.2	0.0	39.2	0.0	0.0	152
Seltzer/club soda (12 fl oz)	0.0	0.0	0.0	0.0	0.0	0
STARBUCKS						
Cappuccino, w/whole milk (12 fl oz)	11.0	0.0	11.0	7.0	7.0	140
Frappuccino, bottled (1 bottle)	37.0	0.0	37.0	7.0	3.5	200
Latte, iced, w/lowfat milk (12 fl oz)	10.0	0.0	10.0	7.0	3.0	90
Latte, iced, w/whole milk (12 fl oz)	10.0	0.0	10.0	6.0	6.0	120
Latte, w/lowfat milk (12 fl oz)	17.0	0.0	17.0	12.0	6.0	170
Latte, w/whole milk (12 fl oz)	17.0	0.0	17.0	11.0	11.0	210
Mocha, w/whole milk (12 fl oz)	33.0	1.0	32.0	12.0	20.0	340
Mocha Frappuccino (12 fl oz)	44.0	0.0	44.0	6.0	3.0	230
TEA						
Brewed (8 fl oz)	0.7	0.0	0.7	0.0	0.0	2
Herbal, brewed (8 fl oz)	0.5	0.0	0.5	0.0	0.0	2
Iced, diet, Nestea (8 fl oz)	1.2	0.0	1.2	0.0	0.0	3

Food Item (Amount)	Carb (g)	Fiber (g)	Net Carbs (g)	Protein (g)	Fat (g)	Cals
Iced, sugar-free, Atkins Lemon Tea Blend (2 tbs)	0.0	0.0	0.0	0.0	0.9	0
Iced, sweetened, Nestea (8 fl oz)	18.0	0.0	18.0	0.0	0.0	65
WATER (8 FL OZ)	0.0	0.0	0.0	0.0	0.0	0

Alcoholic Beverages

BEER

Food Item (Amount)	Carb (g)	Fiber (g)	Net Carbs (g)	Protein (g)	Fat (g)	Cals
Beer (12 fl oz)	13.2	0.7	12.5	1.1	0.0	146
Light (12 fl oz)	4.6	0.0	4.6	0.7	0.0	99
Near (12 fl oz)	5.0	0.0	5.0	1.1	0.0	32
Non-alcoholic, O'Douls (12 fl oz)	15.0	0.0	15.0	0.7	0.0	70
Non-alcoholic, Sharp's (12 fl oz)	12.1	0.0	12.1	0.4	0.0	58

COCKTAILS

Food Item (Amount)	Carb (g)	Fiber (g)	Net Carbs (g)	Protein (g)	Fat (g)	Cals
Bloody Mary (3½ fl oz)	3.3	0.3	3.0	0.5	0.1	77
Margarita (3½ fl oz)	13.9	0.1	13.8	0.1	0.1	219
Pina Colada (3½ fl oz)	24.9	0.4	24.5	0.5	2.1	191
Screwdriver (3½ fl oz)	8.6	0.2	8.5	0.5	0.1	85
HARD LIQUOR (bourbon, gin, rum, vodka, etc., any proof) (1 fl oz)	0.0	0.0	0.0	0.0	0	82
SHERRY, DRY (3½ FL OZ)	1.4	0.0	1.4	0.2	0	72

WINE

Food Item (Amount)	Carb (g)	Fiber (g)	Net Carbs (g)	Protein (g)	Fat (g)	Cals
Dessert, dry (3½ fl oz)	4.2	0.0	4.2	0.2	0	130
Dessert, sweet (3½ fl oz)	12.2	0.0	12.2	0.2	0	158
Non-alcoholic (3½ fl oz)	1.1	0.0	1.1	0.5	0	6
Red (3½ fl oz)	1.8	0.0	1.8	0.2	0	74
White (3½ fl oz)	0.8	0.0	0.8	0.1	0	70
Wine cooler (3½ fl oz)	5.9	0.0	5.9	0.1	0	49

BREADS, MUFFINS AND CRACKERS

It is important to be able to eyeball portions when it comes to breads, muffins and bagels because unit size varies greatly (see pages 19–20). A deli bagel or mega-muffin can easily pack a day's worth of carbs. The best choices are controlled carbohydrate baked goods. When they aren't available, opt for multigrain or whole wheat breads in slices about the size of your palm. Before eating crackers or breadsticks, separate the number you want to eat, then put the package away. When you've finished your allotment, don't reach for more. (This is a good way to prevent mindless munching). Toast bread whenever possible—crunchy food takes longer to chew. And once you're in the Lifetime Maintenance phase and choose to eat conventional bread, opt for open-faced sandwiches instead of standard ones.

Food Item (Amount)	Carb (g)	Fiber (g)	Net Carbs (g)	Protein (g)	Fat (g)	Cals
Bagel						
Atkins, plain (1/2 bagel)	12.0	6.0	6.0	9.0	3.0	90
Cinnamon Raisin (41/2")	65.1	2.7	62.4	11.6	2.0	323
Plain (31/2")	37.9	1.6	36.3	7.5	1.1	195
Plain, poppy, sesame (41/2")	58.7	2.5	56.2	11.6	1.8	303
Biscuit						
Homemade (21/2")	26.8	0.9	25.9	4.2	9.8	212
Gold Medal (1)	22.0	0.5	21.5	3.0	7.0	160
Grands (1)	25.0	0.8	24.3	4.0	9.0	200
Hungry Jack Refrigerated Fluffy (1)	11.4	0.4	11.0	1.7	4.1	89
Pillsbury Buttermilk Refrigerated (1)	30.4	0.0	30.4	5.0	1.4	154
Bread						
ATKINS BREAD						
Country White (1 slice)	7.0	4.0	3.0	7.0	2.0	70
Traditional Rye (1 slice)	7.0	4.0	3.0	7.0	2.0	70
ATKINS BREAD MIX						
Quick and Easy Caraway Rye (1 slice)	8.0	5.0	3.0	12.0	2.7	95
Quick and Easy Country White (1 slice)	8.0	5.0	3.0	12.0	2.7	95
Quick and Easy Sourdough (1 slice)	8.0	5.0	3.0	12.0	2.7	95
BREADSTICK						
Brown & serve (1)	28.0	1.0	27.0	7.0	1.5	150
Sesame (1 small)	2.0	0.0	2.0	0.0	0.0	15
Cornbread (21/2" square)	22.7	1.9	20.7	4.0	4.9	152

Food Item (Amount)	Carb (g)	Fiber (g)	Net Carbs (g)	Protein (g)	Fat (g)	Cals
French (1-oz slice)	14.7	0.9	13.9	2.5	0.9	78
Italian (1-oz slice)	14.2	0.8	13.4	2.5	1.0	77
Oatmeal (1-oz slice)	13.8	1.1	12.6	2.4	1.3	76
Pita, white (6½" diameter)	33.4	1.3	32.1	5.5	0.7	165
Pita, whole wheat (6½" diameter)	35.2	4.7	30.5	6.3	1.7	170
Pumpernickel (1-oz slice)	13.5	1.8	11.6	2.5	0.9	71
Raisin (1-oz slice)	14.8	1.2	13.6	2.2	1.3	78
Rye (1-oz slice)	13.7	1.6	12.1	2.4	0.9	73
Sourdough (1-oz slice)	14.7	0.9	13.9	2.5	0.9	78
Wheat (1-oz slice)	13.4	1.2	12.2	2.6	1.2	74
White (1-oz slice)	14.0	0.7	13.4	2.3	1.0	76
Whole grain (1-oz slice)	13.4	1.2	12.2	2.6	1.2	74
Crackers						
100% Stoned Wheat (3)	8.2	1.2	7.0	1.1	2.1	53
Bran-a-Crisp (1)	6.0	2.0	4.0	1.0	0.0	20
Brown rice snaps (8)	11.0	1.0	10.0	1.0	0.0	50
Cheez-It (12)	7.5	0.4	7.1	1.8	3.9	72
Crispbread						
Finn Crisp (3)	11.0	3.0	8.0	2.0	0.0	60
Kavli Crispy Thin (3)	13.0	2.0	11.0	1.0	0.0	60
Ryvita Flavorful Fiber (2)	14.0	3.0	11.0	2.0	0.0	60
Wasa Hearty Rye (1)	9.0	2.0	7.0	1.0	0.0	45
DLIGHTFUL BAKERY						
Sesame (2)	4.0	0.0	4.0	0.0	3.0	50
Whole Wheat (2)	4.0	0.0	4.0	0.0	3.0	50
FLATBREAD						
JJ Flats (1)	9.0	1.0	8.0	2.0	2.0	60

Food Item (Amount)	Carb (g)	Fiber (g)	Net Carbs (g)	Protein (g)	Fat (g)	Cals
Nejaimes Lavash (1/2)	10.0	1.0	9.0	2.0	2.0	70
Harvest Crisp 5-Grain (13)	23.0	1.0	22.0	3.0	3.5	130
HEALTH VALLEY						
Sesame, low fat (5)	10.0	1.0	9.0	2.0	1.5	60
Stoned Wheat, low fat (5)	10.0	1.0	9.0	2.0	1.0	60
Matzoh, plain (1/2)	11.8	0.4	11.4	1.4	0.2	56
Melba toast (2)	7.7	0.6	7.0	1.2	0.3	39
Rite Lite Rounds, Barbara's (5)	12.0	0.0	12.0	1.0	<1.0	55
Ritz (5)	10.0	0.0	10.0	1.0	4.0	80
Saltines (5)	10.8	0.4	10.4	1.4	1.8	65
Teriyaki Brown Rice, San-J (3)	13.0	0.5	12.5	1.5	0.5	60
Town House (4)	8.3	0.3	8.0	1.0	4.2	75
Triscuit (3)	9.0	1.3	7.7	1.3	2.6	64
Uneeda Biscuits (2)	10.5	0.2	10.3	1.5	1.5	65
Water Biscuit, Pepperidge Farm (4)	11.4	0.0	11.4	1.7	1.3	61
Water Biscuit, Carr's (5)	13.0	1.0	12.0	2.0	1.5	70
Wheat Thins (8)	10.0	0.4	9.6	1.2	5.9	68
Wheatsworth (5)	10.0	1.0	9.0	2.0	3.5	80
Whole Wheat, Carr's (2)	11.0	1.0	10.0	1.0	3.5	80
Zweiback (1)	6.0	0.0	6.0	1.0	1.0	35
English Muffin						
Cinnamon raisin (1)	27.8	1.7	26.1	4.3	1.5	139
Plain (1)	26.2	1.5	24.7	4.4	1.0	134
Sourdough (1)	25.8	1.5	24.3	4.3	1.0	132
Whole wheat (1)	26.7	4.4	22.2	5.8	1.4	134

Food Item (Amount)	Carb (g)	Fiber (g)	Net Carbs (g)	Protein (g)	Fat (g)	Cals
Garlic Bread						
Pepperidge Farm (1)	14.0	1.0	13.0	5.0	10.0	160
Muffin (2 oz)						
ATKINS MUFFIN MIX						
Banana Nut (1)	6.0	4.0	2.0	8.0	2.0	70
Chocolate Chocolate Chip (1)	16.0	5.0	6.0	8.0	1.0	90
Corn (1)	7.0	4.0	3.0	9.0	0.5	60
Lemon Poppy (1)	7.0	4.0	3.0	9.0	1.0	60
Orange Cranberry (1)	7.0	4.0	3.0	9.0	0.5	60
Banana nut (1)	29.0	1.0	28.0	3.0	7.0	190
Blueberry (1)	27.2	1.5	25.8	3.1	3.7	157
Blueberry, toaster (1)	17.6	0.6	17.0	1.5	3.1	103
Bran (1)	23.7	4.0	19.7	4.0	7.3	163
Corn (1)	28.9	1.9	26.9	3.4	4.8	173
Roll						
Crescent, Pillsbury, refrigerated (1)	11.0	0.0	11.0	2.0	6.0	110
Croissant, Sara Lee Original (1)	20.0	1.0	19.0	4.0	8.0	170
Dinner, Brown & Serve (1 oz)	14.3	0.9	13.4	2.4	2.1	85
Hamburger (1½ oz)	21.7	1.3	20.4	3.6	3.1	129
White, hard (1 oz)	14.9	0.7	14.3	2.8	1.2	83
Whole wheat (1 oz)	14.5	2.1	12.4	2.5	1.3	75
Stuffing						
Cornbread, Stove Top (½ cup)	19.0	1.0	18.0	3.0	8.0	160
Turkey, Stove Top (½ cup)	20.0	1.0	19.0	4.0	9.0	170

Food Item (Amount)	Carb (g)	Fiber (g)	Net Carbs (g)	Protein (g)	Fat (g)	Cals
Tortillas						
La Tortilla Factory, all flavors (1)	12.0	9.0	3.0	5.0	2.0	60
Corn (1)	12.1	1.4	10.7	1.5	0.6	58
Flour (1)	27.2	1.6	25.6	4.3	3.5	159
Whole wheat (1)	20.0	1.9	18.1	2.9	0.4	73

CEREALS AND CEREAL BARS

Fiber counts here, because it accounts for the major differences in grams of Net Carbs. Therefore, when you are on Pre-Maintenance and Lifetime Maintenance, opt for fiber-rich whole grain products with no added sugar. (The less said about multi-colored puffed cereal coated with sugar, the better!) The counts given are for half-cup servings: Not very big amounts for a lot of carbs—so add cereals only when you are near your goal weight. A better option is to only eat controlled carb products. Most cereal bars contain sugar, and should be avoided.

Food Item (Amount).	Carb (g)	Fiber (g)	Net Carbs (g)	Protein (g)	Fat (g)	Cals

Cereal

CEREAL, HOT, COOKED

Food Item (Amount).	Carb (g)	Fiber (g)	Net Carbs (g)	Protein (g)	Fat (g)	Cals
..Atkins Hot Cereal (1/2 cup)	10.0	4.5	5.6	10.0	1.0	80
Cream of Rice (1/2 cup)	13.9	0.1	13.8	1.1	0.1	63
Cream of Wheat, instant, prepared w/water (1/2 cup)	15.8	1.5	14.3	2.2	0.2	77
Cream of Wheat, flavored, (1 packet)	29.0	0.5	28.5	2.4	0.5	132
Farina (1/2 cup)	12.4	1.6	10.7	1.6	0.1	58
Grits (1/2 cup)	15.7	0.2	15.5	1.7	0.2	73
Maltex (1/2 cup)	19.8	1.5	18.3	2.9	0.5	90
OATMEAL						
Cinnamon Spice (1 packet)	35.9	3.0	32.9	3.9	2.1	172
Blueberry & Cream (1 packet)	26.1	2.0	24.1	2.7	2.7	135
Instant (1 packet)	18.1	3.1	15.1	4.4	1.7	105
Plain (all cuts of oats) (1/2 cup)	12.6	2.0	10.7	3.0	1.2	73
Wheatena (1/2 cup)	14.3	3.3	11.1	2.4	0.6	68
CEREAL, READY-TO-EAT:						
All-Bran (1/2 cup)	23.5	10.0	13.5	3.8	1.0	82
Apple Jacks (1/2 cup)	14.8	0.3	14.5	0.8	0.2	64
Atkins Cereal (1/2 cup)	9.0	5.0	4.0	16.0	3.3	116
Atkins Cereal with Almonds (1/2 cup)	9.0	5.0	4.0	18.0	0.5	132
Bran Buds (1/2 cup)	36.3	18.1	18.2	4.3	1.1	125
Cheerios (1/2 cup)	8.6	1.0	7.6	1.2	0.7	41
Cheerios, Multigrain (1/2 cup)	12.2	1.0	11.3	1.3	0.5	56
Cocoa Puffs (1/2 cup)	13.4	0.1	13.3	0.6	0.5	59
Complete Bran Flakes (1/2 cup)	15.4	3.1	12.4	2.0	0.4	63

Food Item (Amount)	Carb (g)	Fiber (g)	Net Carbs (g)	Protein (g)	Fat (g)	Cals
Corn Chex (1/2 cup)	12.1	0.3	11.8	1.0	0.2	53
Corn Flakes (1/2 cup)	12.1	0.4	11.7	0.9	0.1	51
Cracklin' Oat Bran (1/2 cup)	23.8	3.9	19.9	2.7	4.1	134
Crispix (1/2 cup)	12.5	0.3	12.2	1.1	0.1	54
Fiber One (1/2 cup)	24.0	14.3	9.8	2.8	0.8	62
Frosted Flakes (1/2 cup)	18.9	0.4	18.4	0.8	0.1	80
Frosted Mini Wheats (1/2 cup)	22.7	2.9	19.8	2.6	0.4	93
Froot Loops (1/2 cup)	14.1	0.3	13.8	0.8	0.5	63
Granola (1/2 cup)	20.5	2.0	18.5	4.5	5.5	150
Grape Nuts Flakes (1/2 cup)	15.8	1.7	14.1	1.9	0.6	71
Kashi, Honey Puffed (1/2 cup)	12.5	1.0	11.5	1.5	0.5	60
Kashi, Puffed (1/2 cup)	6.5	1.0	5.5	1.5	0.5	35
Kashi Medley (1/2 cup)	20.0	2.0	18.0	4.0	1.0	100
Kix (1/2 cup)	8.2	0.3	7.9	0.6	0.2	36
Life (1/2 cup)	17.3	1.4	15.9	2.2	0.9	83
Mother's Harvest Oat Flake (1/2 cup)	15.6	1.5	14.1	1.8	0.8	73
Nut & Honey Crunch (1/2 cup)	15.3	0.3	15.0	1.3	0.8	74
Nutlettes All-In-One-Cereal (1/3 cup)	12.0	7.0	5.0	25.0	2.0	133
Oatmeal Squares (1/2 cup)	21.7	2.1	19.5	3.6	1.3	108
Organic Soy Essence (1/2 cup)	16.8	3.4	13.4	2.0	0.3	67
Product 19 (1/2 cup)	12.5	0.5	12.0	1.3	0.2	55
Protein Crunch Plain (1/3 cup)	6.0	1.0	5.0	26.0	4.0	170
Puffed Rice (1/2 cup)	6.3	0.1	6.2	0.4	0.0	28
Raisin Bran (1/2 cup)	23.6	4.1	19.5	2.8	0.7	93
Rice Krispies (1/2 cup)	11.4	0.2	11.3	0.8	0.2	50
Shredded Spoonfuls (1/2 cup)	16.0	2.7	13.3	2.7	1.0	80

Food Item (Amount)	Carb (g)	Fiber (g)	Net Carbs (g)	Protein (g)	Fat (g)	Cals
Shredded Wheat, large biscuit (2 biscuits)	38.4	4.6	33.7	5.1	0.8	170
Shredded Wheat, small biscuit (1/2 cup)	17.2	2.1	15.1	2.4	0.4	76
Special K (1/2 cup)	11.2	0.5	10.7	3.2	0.1	57
Spelt Flakes (1/2 cup)	11.0	1.5	9.5	2.5	0.5	50
Puffed Wheat (1/2 cup)	10.0	1.0	9.0	1.5	0.3	45
Total Wheat (1/2 cup)	15.9	1.8	14.2	2.0	0.5	70
Trix (1/2 cup)	12.2	0.3	11.8	0.5	0.8	57
Wheaties (1/2 cup)	11.5	1.0	10.5	1.6	0.5	53
Cereal Bars						
Chocolate-Coated Granola (1)	22.7	1.2	21.5	2.2	7.3	158
Nature's Choice Carob Chip Granola (1)	16.0	2.0	14.0	2.0	2.0	80
Nutri Grain Strawberry (1)	27.0	1.0	26.0	2.0	3.0	140
Peanut Butter Granola (1)	14.7	0.7	14.0	2.3	5.6	114
Snackwell's Blueberry (1)	29.3	1.2	28.1	1.0	0.3	121

PANCAKES, WAFFLES AND BREAKFAST PASTRIES

Controlled carbohydrate pancake mix and French toast made from Atkins bread are two smart choices when you don't want eggs for breakfast. Commercial breakfast pastries—even those weighing a scant 2 ounces—are made with white flour, sugar and sweet fillings—and all are loaded with carbs. The best advice we can give you is to stay away from them.

Food Item (Amount)	Carb (g)	Fiber (g)	Net Carbs (g)	Protein (g)	Fat (g)	Cals
Breakfast Pastries						
Atkins Creamy Cinnamon Bun Breakfast Bar (1)	2.0	1.0	1.0	12.0	8.0	150
CINNAMON ROLL						
Pepperidge Farm (1)	33.0	2.0	31.0	4.0	12.0	250
Pillsbury w/Icing, refrigerated (1)	23.9	0.0	23.9	2.4	5.0	150
Pillsbury Sweet Rolls, frozen (1)	53.0	1.0	52.0	6.0	10.0	330
Coffeecake, crumb topping (2 oz)	29.4	1.3	28.2	4.3	14.7	263
DANISH						
Cinnamon (2 oz)	25.3	0.7	24.6	4.0	12.7	229
Entenmann's, Pecan Pastry Ring (2 oz)	24.6	1.1	23.5	3.2	16.1	246
Pepperidge Farm Cheese (2 oz)	21.8	0.9	20.9	5.2	9.6	201
DOUGHNUT						
Apple fritter, Dunkin Donuts (1)	41.0	2.0	39.0	5.0	13.0	300
Bow Tie, Dunkin Donuts (1)	35.0	1.0	34.0	5.0	10.0	250
Cake (1)	23.4	0.7	22.7	2.4	10.8	198
Chocolate Cake, Dunkin Donuts (1)	19.0	1.0	18.0	3.0	14.0	210
Glazed Yeast (1)	26.6	0.7	25.9	3.8	13.7	242
FRENCH TOAST						
Aunt Jemima, frozen (1 slice)	13.3	0.7	12.6	3.4	2.2	83
Homemade (2-oz piece)	16.3	0.6	15.7	5.0	7.0	149
Pepperidge Farm, frozen (1 slice)	23.0	1.0	22.0	5.0	5.0	160

Food Item (Amount)	Carb (g)	Fiber (g)	Net Carbs (g)	Protein (g)	Fat (g)	Cals
Pancakes						
Atkins Pancake & Waffle Mix (1)	2.0	1.0	1.0	3.4	3.0	52
Blueberry, Aunt Jemima (1)	15.5	0.4	15.1	2.3	1.3	83
From mix (1)	22.3	1.4	20.8	6.0	5.9	168
Frozen (6-inch)	31.8	1.3	30.5	3.8	2.4	167
Pancakes with Sausage, Great Start (1 pkg)	52.0	3.0	49.0	14.0	25.0	490
Toaster Pastry						
Frosted PopTart (1)	37.4	0.5	36.9	2.2	5.3	204
Health Valley Low Fat Fruit Tart (1)	28.0	1.0	27.0	2.0	2.0	130
Pop Tart (1)	32.2	0.8	31.5	2.7	9.2	219
Toaster Strudel Pastry, Cream Cheese, frozen (1)	23.0	0.5	22.5	3.0	11.0	200
Waffles						
Atkins Pancake & Waffle Mix (1)	2.0	1.0	1.0	3.4	3.0	52
Aunt Jemima Blueberry (1)	14.6	0.6	14.0	2.1	2.6	88
Eggo Buttermilk (1)	15.0	0.0	15.0	2.5	4.0	110
Hungry Jack Homestyle (1)	14.5	0.5	14.0	1.5	3.0	90

FRUIT

Berries are the preferred fruit on Atkins, because of their high fiber content and relatively low carb count. Keep portion size in mind though (see pages 19–20), because a half-cup of berries—the recommended quantity—is a small amount. One trick to make berries last longer is to pop them in the freezer and eat them partially frozen. Kiwi fruit is another good option; it's loaded with vitamins and contains only 8.7 grams of Net Carbs per fruit. Rhubarb, which needs to be cooked, is an often overlooked choice. It is excellent when prepared with sugar substitute and lemon peel. Dried fruits, such as raisins, prunes and dates are much higher in carbs than their fresh counterparts. Keep in mind that whole fruit is always a better choice than fruit juice, which is higher in carbs and missing all or much of the fiber.

Food Item (Amount)	Carb (g)	Fiber (g)	Net Carbs (g)	Protein (g)	Fat (g)	Cals
Acerola (1/2 cup)	3.8	0.5	3.2	0.2	0.2	16
Apple (1/2 medium)	10.5	1.9	8.7	0.1	0.3	41
APPLESAUCE						
Sweetened (1/2 cup)	25.4	1.5	23.9	0.2	0.2	97
Unsweetened (1/2 cup)	13.8	1.5	12.3	0.2	0.1	52
APRICOTS						
Canned, in juice (3 halves)	13.3	1.7	11.6	0.7	0.0	52
Dried, (6 halves)	13.0	1.9	11.1	0.8	0.1	50
Fresh (3 whole)	11.7	2.5	9.2	1.5	0.4	50
AVOCADO						
California (Haas) (1/2)	6.0	4.2	1.7	1.8	15.0	153
Florida (1/2)	13.5	8.1	5.5	2.4	13.5	170
Banana, small (1)	23.7	2.4	21.2	1.0	0.5	93
Banana chips (1/4 cup)	13.4	1.8	11.7	0.5	7.7	119
BLACKBERRIES						
Fresh (1/2 cup)	9.2	3.8	5.4	0.5	0.3	37
Frozen, unsweetened (1/2 cup)	11.8	3.8	8.1	0.9	0.3	48
BLUEBERRIES						
Fresh (1/2 cup)	10.2	2.0	8.3	0.5	0.3	41
Frozen, sweetened (1/2 cup)	25.2	2.4	22.8	0.5	0.2	93
Frozen, unsweetened (1/2 cup)	9.4	2.1	7.4	0.3	0.5	40
BOYSENBERRIES						
Fresh (1/2 cup)	9.2	3.8	5.4	0.5	0.3	37
Frozen, unsweetened (1/2 cup)	8.1	2.6	5.5	0.7	0.2	33
Cherimoya (1/2 cup)	27.0	2.7	24.3	1.5	0.5	106
CHERRIES						
Sour, canned, in water (1/2 cup)	10.9	1.3	9.6	0.9	0.1	44
Sour, fresh (1/2 cup)	6.3	0.8	5.5	0.5	0.2	26

Food Item (Amount)	Carb (g)	Fiber (g)	Net Carbs (g)	Protein (g)	Fat (g)	Cals
Sweet, canned, in water (1/2 cup)	14.6	1.9	12.7	1.0	0.2	57
Sweet, fresh (1/2 cup)	9.7	1.3	8.3	0.7	0.6	42
Cranberries, raw, no sugar (1/2 cup)	6.0	2.0	4.0	0.2	0.1	23
DATES						
Chopped (1/2 cup)	65.4	6.7	58.8	1.8	0.4	245
Fresh (3)	18.3	1.9	16.4	0.5	0.1	68
FIGS						
Canned, in water (1/2 cup)	17.4	2.7	14.6	0.5	0.1	66
Fresh, small (1)	7.7	1.3	6.4	0.3	0.1	30
FRUIT COCKTAIL						
Canned, in heavy syrup (1/2 cup)	23.5	1.2	22.2	0.5	0.1	91
Canned, in water (1/2 cup)	10.1	1.2	8.9	0.5	0.1	38
FRUIT SALAD						
Canned, in heavy syrup (1/2 cup)	24.4	1.3	23.1	0.4	0.1	93
Canned, in juice (1/2 cup)	16.3	1.3	15.0	0.6	0.0	62
Gooseberries, raw, no sugar (1/2 cup)	7.6	3.2	4.4	0.7	0.4	33
GRAPEFRUIT						
Fresh (1/2 cup)	9.5	1.7	7.8	0.7	0.1	37
Sections (1/2 cup)	9.3	1.3	8.0	0.7	0.1	37
GRAPES						
Green seedless (1/2 cup)	14.2	0.8	13.4	0.5	0.5	57
Slip skin (purple Concord) (1/2 cup)	7.9	0.5	7.4	0.3	0.2	31

Food Item (Amount)	Carb (g)	Fiber (g)	Net Carbs (g)	Protein (g)	Fat (g)	Cals
Tokay/Empress/RedFlame (red seedless) (1/2 cup)	14.2	0.8	13.4	0.5	0.5	57
Guava (1/2 cup)	9.8	4.5	5.3	0.7	0.5	42
Guava paste (2 tbs)	20.6	0.3	20.3	0.0	0.0	80
JUICES (see Beverages-nonalcoholic)						
Kiwifruit (1)	11.3	2.6	8.7	0.8	0.3	46
Kumquat (4)	12.5	5.0	7.5	0.7	0.1	48
Lemon juice (2 tbs)	2.6	0.1	2.5	0.1	0.0	8
Loganberries (1/2 cup)	9.2	3.8	5.4	0.5	0.3	37
Loquat, small (10)	16.5	2.3	14.2	0.6	0.3	64
LYCHEES						
Fresh (1/2 cup)	15.7	1.2	14.5	0.8	0.4	63
Fresh, whole (10)	15.9	1.3	14.6	0.8	0.4	63
MANGO						
Dried (1 piece)	8.0	0.0	8.0	0.0	0.3	33
Fresh (1/2 cup)	14.0	1.5	12.5	0.4	0.2	54
MELON						
Cantaloupe						
Balls (1/2 cup)	7.4	0.7	6.7	0.8	0.3	31
Medium (5" diameter, 1/2)	23.1	2.2	20.9	2.4	0.8	97
Crenshaw melon, balls (1/2 cup)	5.3	0.7	4.6	0.8	0.1	22
Honeydew, balls (1/2 cup)	7.8	0.5	7.3	0.4	0.1	30
Watermelon, balls (1/2 cup)	5.5	0.4	5.1	0.5	0.3	25
Nectarine (1)	16.0	2.2	13.8	1.3	0.6	67
ORANGE						
Sections (1/2 cup)	10.6	2.2	8.4	0.9	0.1	42
Whole (1)	16.3	3.4	12.9	1.4	0.1	64

Food Item (Amount)	Carb (g)	Fiber (g)	Net Carbs (g)	Protein (g)	Fat (g)	Cals
PAPAYA						
Dried (1 piece)	14.9	2.7	12.2	0.9	0.2	59
Fresh, small (1/2)	7.5	1.4	6.1	0.5	0.1	30
Passion Fruit (1/4 cup)	13.8	6.1	7.7	1.3	0.4	57
PEACH						
Canned, in water (1/2 cup)	7.5	1.6	5.9	0.5	0.1	29
Dried, halves (2)	16.0	2.1	13.8	0.9	0.2	62
Fresh, small (1)	8.8	1.6	7.2	0.6	0.1	34
PEAR						
Canned in water, halves (1/2 cup)	9.5	2.0	7.6	0.2	0.0	35
Fresh, medium, Bartlett (1)	25.1	4.0	21.1	0.7	0.7	98
Fresh, small, Bosc (1)	21.0	3.3	17.7	0.5	0.6	82
Persimmon, large (1/2)	15.6	3.0	12.6	0.5	0.2	59
PINEAPPLE						
Canned, in water (1/2 cup)	10.2	1.0	9.2	0.5	0.1	39
Fresh, chunks (1/2 cup)	9.6	0.9	8.7	0.3	0.3	38
PLUM						
Dried (prune) (4)	21.1	2.4	18.7	0.9	0.2	80
Dried (prune), canned, in heavy syrup (1/2 cup)	32.5	4.5	28.1	1.0	0.2	123
Fresh, small (1)	3.7	0.4	3.3	0.2	0.2	16
Purple, canned, in water (1/2 cup)	13.7	1.3	12.5	0.5	0.0	51
Pomegranate (1/4)	6.6	0.2	6.4	0.4	0.1	26
RAISINS						
Golden (1 tbs)	8.2	0.4	7.8	0.4	0.0	31
Seedless (1 tbs)	8.1	0.7	7.4	0.3	0.1	31

Food Item (Amount)	Carb (g)	Fiber (g)	Net Carbs (g)	Protein (g)	Fat (g)	Cals
RASPBERRIES						
Fresh (1/2 cup)	7.1	4.2	3.0	0.6	0.3	30
Frozen, sweetened (1/2 cup)	32.7	5.5	27.2	0.9	0.2	129
Rhubarb, fresh (1/2 cup)	2.8	1.1	1.7	0.6	0.1	13
STRAWBERRIES						
Fresh, whole (1/2 cup)	5.1	1.7	3.4	0.4	0.3	22
Frozen, sweetened (1/2 cup)	33.0	2.4	30.6	0.7	0.2	122
Frozen, unsweetened (1/2 cup)	6.8	1.6	5.2	0.3	0.1	26
Tangerine, small (1)	7.8	1.6	6.2	0.4	0.1	31

EGGS AND CHEESE

Most hard cheeses are full fat, low in carbs and can be enjoyed on all phases of Atkins. You can eat fresh cheeses, such as ricotta and cottage cheese, after Induction. Be leery of "cheese products" and "cheese spreads" because they are higher in carbs and often highly processed. Serving size counts here: Cheese is a dense food. One ounce of hard cheese is really small—about the size of a pair of dice. Add volume to cheese by shredding it—2 ounces shredded is about a half-cup.

Food Item (Amount)	Carb (g)	Fiber (g)	Net Carbs (g)	Protein (g)	Fat (g)	Cals
Eggs						
Fried (1)	0.6	0.0	0.6	6.2	6.9	92
Poached/boiled (1)	0.6	0.0	0.6	6.3	5.3	78
QUICHE, ATKINS, HEAT & SERVE						
Bacon & Onion Crustless (1)	2.0	0.0	2.0	18.0	27.0	320
Four Cheese Crustless (1)	2.0	0.0	2.0	22.0	24.0	290
Smoked Ham & Cheese Crustless (1)	2.0	0.0	2.0	18.0	24.0	290
Scrambled, with milk (1)	1.3	0.0	1.3	6.8	7.5	101
Scrambled, egg substitute (1/4 cup)	1.4	0.0	1.4	3.6	4.1	58
SOUFFLE, ATKINS, HEAT & SERVE						
Broccoli, Cheddar, Bacon (1)	3.0	0.0	3.0	12.0	15.0	200
Crab & Cheddar (1)	2.0	0.0	2.0	13.0	25.0	290
Spinach, Tomato & Feta (1)	4.0	2.0	2.0	10.0	13.0	170
White, before cooking (1/4 cup)	0.6	0.0	0.6	6.0	0.0	29
Cheese						
American Cheese (1 slice, 2/3 oz)	0.3	0.0	0.3	4.7	6.6	79
American Cheese Food (1 slice, 2/3 oz)	1.5	0.0	1.5	4.1	5.2	69
Blue, crumbled (2 tbs)	0.4	0.0	0.4	3.6	4.9	60
Boursin (2 tbs)	1.0	0.0	1.0	2.0	13.0	120
Brie (1 oz)	0.1	0.0	0.1	5.9	7.9	95
Camembert (1 oz)	0.1	0.0	0.1	5.6	6.9	85
Cheddar (1 oz)	0.4	0.0	0.4	7.1	9.4	114
Cheez Whiz (2 tbs)	3.0	0.1	2.9	4.0	6.9	91
Cottage, 2% fat (1/2 cup)	4.1	0.0	4.1	15.5	2.2	101
Cottage, creamed (1/2 cup)	2.8	0.0	2.8	13.1	4.7	109
Cracker Barrel (2 tbs)	4.0	0.0	4.0	5.0	8.0	100

Food Item (Amount)	Carb (g)	Fiber (g)	Net Carbs (g)	Protein (g)	Fat (g)	Cals
CREAM						
Chive & Onion (2 tbs)	2.0	0.0	2.0	2.0	10.0	110
Plain (2 tbs)	0.8	0.0	0.8	2.2	10.1	101
Strawberry (2 tbs)	5.0	0.0	5.0	1.0	9.0	100
Edam (1 oz)	0.4	0.0	0.4	7.1	7.9	101
Feta (1 oz)	1.2	0.0	1.2	4.0	6.0	75
Fontina (1 oz)	0.4	0.0	0.4	7.3	8.8	110
Goat, soft (1 oz)	0.3	0.0	0.3	5.3	6.0	76
Gorgonzola (1 oz)	0.0	0.0	0.0	7.0	9.0	111
Gouda (1 oz)	0.6	0.0	0.6	7.1	7.8	101
Havarti (1 oz)	0.8	0.0	0.8	6.6	8.4	105
Jarlsberg (1 oz)	1.0	0.0	1.0	8.1	7.8	107
Laughing Cow (1 wedge)	1.0	0.0	1.0	2.0	4.0	50
Mascarpone (1 oz)	0.6	0.0	0.6	2.0	13.2	126
Mozzarella, whole milk (1 oz)	0.6	0.0	0.6	5.5	6.1	80
Mozzarella, part skim (1 oz)	0.8	0.0	0.8	6.9	4.5	72
Muenster (1 oz)	0.3	0.0	0.3	6.6	8.5	104
Neuchatel (2 tbs)	2.0	0.0	2.0	3.0	5.0	70
Parmesan, chunk (1 oz)	0.9	0.0	0.9	10.1	7.3	111
Parmesan, grated (1 tbs)	0.2	0.0	0.2	2.6	1.9	28
Port Wine spread (2 tbs)	4.5	0.0	4.5	4.5	5.6	90
Provolone (1 oz)	0.6	0.0	0.6	7.3	7.6	100
Ricotta, whole milk (1/4 cup)	1.9	0.0	1.9	6.9	8.0	107
Ricotta, part skim (1/4 cup)	3.2	0.0	3.2	7.0	4.9	85
Romano, chunk (1 oz)	1.0	0.0	1.0	9.1	7.1	105
Romano, grated (1 tbs)	0.2	0.0	0.2	2.0	1.7	24
Swiss (1 oz)	1.0	0.0	1.0	8.1	7.8	107
Swiss Knight (1 wedge)	0.0	0.0	0.0	6.0	6.0	82
Velveeta (1 oz)	2.8	0.0	2.8	4.6	6.2	86

MILK, CREAM, BUTTER AND YOGURT

Most low-fat yogurts (and there are a zillion of them) are high in carbohydrates. For a much lower-carb—and better tasting—fruit yogurt, buy whole milk yogurt, sweeten it with sugar substitute and mix in chopped berries. As for sour cream and heavy cream, note that the carb count given is for small amounts (2 tablespoons and 1 tablespoon respectively), so keep that in mind when topping vegetables or adding cream to your decaf coffee.

Food Item (Amount)	Carb (g)	Fiber (g)	Net Carbs (g)	Protein (g)	Fat (g)	Cals
Butter						
Butter (1 tbs)	0.0	0.0	0.0	0.1	11.5	102
Butter, whipped (1 tbs)	0.0	0.0	0.0	0.0	7.0	70
Cream						
Half and Half (1 tbs)	0.5	0.0	0.5	0.5	1.5	20
Heavy, liquid (1 tbs)	0.4	0.0	0.4	0.3	5.5	51
Heavy, whipped (2 tbs)	0.4	0.0	0.4	0.3	5.5	52
Light (1 tbs)	0.6	0.0	0.6	0.4	2.9	29
CREAMER, NONDAIRY						
Coffeemate Fat Free Hazelnut (1 tbs)	5.0	0.0	5.0	0.0	0.0	25
Coffeemate Flavored (1 tbs)	5.0	0.0	5.0	0.0	2.0	40
Coffeemate Plain (1 tbs)	2.0	0.0	2.0	0.0	1.0	20
Milk						
BUTTERMILK,						
Cultured from 1% milk (1 cup)	13.0	0.0	13.0	9.0	2.5	110
Cultured from skim milk (1 cup)	11.7	0.0	11.7	8.1	2.2	99
Condensed, canned (2 tbs)	20.8	0.0	20.8	3.0	3.3	123
Evaporated, 2% (2 tbs)	3.5	0.0	3.5	2.3	0.6	29
Evaporated, whole (2 tbs)	3.2	0.0	3.2	2.2	2.4	42
Lowfat (1%) (1 cup)	11.7	0.0	11.7	8.0	2.6	102
Nonfat (skim) (1 cup)	11.9	0.0	11.9	8.4	0.4	86
Reduced fat, 2% (1 cup)	11.7	0.0	11.7	8.1	4.7	121
Whole (1 cup)	11.4	0.0	11.4	8.0	8.2	150
FLAVORED MILK						
(See Beverages, nonalcoholic)						
RICE MILK						
Plain (1 cup)	25.0	0.0	25.0	1.0	2.0	120

Food Item (Amount)	Carb (g)	Fiber (g)	Net Carbs (g)	Protein (g)	Fat (g)	Cals
Vanilla (1 cup)	28.0	0.0	28.0	1.0	2.0	130
SOY MILK						
Chocolate, Soy Dream (8 fl oz)	37.0	1.0	36.0	7.0	3.5	210
Light, Vitasoy (8 fl oz)	15.0	0.0	15.0	4.0	2.0	90
Plain (8 fl oz)	4.4	3.2	1.2	6.7	4.7	81
Vanilla, Soy Dream (8 fl oz)	22.0	0.0	22.0	7.0	4.0	150
Sour Cream						
Light (2 tbs)	2.0	0.0	2.0	2.0	2.5	40
Regular (2 tbs)	1.2	0.0	1.2	0.9	6.0	62
Yogurt						
BREYERS						
Blueberry Lowfat (8 oz)	48.0	0.0	48.0	8.0	2.5	250
Coffee, Lemon, or Vanilla Lowfat (8 oz)	38.0	0.0	38.0	10.0	3.0	220
Strawberry Lowfat (8 oz)	41.3	0.5	40.8	8.6	1.8	218
COLOMBO						
Classic (8 oz)	42.0	0.0	42.0	7.0	2.0	220
Light (8 oz)	21.0	0.0	21.0	7.0	1.0	120
DANNON						
Blended Snack Packs (4 oz)	20-21	0.0	20-21	5.0	0.0	100
Flavored (8 oz)	36-37	0.0	36-37	11.0	3.5	220-230
Fruit on the Bottom (8 oz)	39-44	0.1	39-44	9.0	2-3	210-240
Frusion (10 oz)	51-53	0.0	51-53	8.0	3.5	270
la Crème (4 oz)	20.0	0.0	20.0	5.0	5.0	140
Lite 'n Fit (8 oz)	21-24	0.0	21-24	8.0	0.0	120
PLAIN						
Lowfat (8 oz)	15.0	0.0	15.0	11.0	3.0	130
Whole milk (8 fl oz)	11.0	0.0	11.0	9.0	8.0	150

Food Item (Amount)	Carb (g)	Fiber (g)	Net Carbs (g)	Protein (g)	Fat (g)	Cals
STONYFIELD FARM						
Nonfat Raspberry (8 oz)	31.0	1.0	30.0	8.0	0.0	160
Whole Milk Vanilla (6 oz)	37.0	0.0	37.0	7.0	5.0	220
YOPLAIT						
Custard (6 oz)	32.0	0.0	32.0	7.0	3.5	190
Expresse (1)	11.0	0.0	11.0	2.0	1.5	70
Light (6 oz)	19.0	0.0	19.0	5-6	0.0	100
Original (6 oz)	33.0	0.0	33.0	5	1.5	170

SWEETENERS, JAMS AND SYRUPS

Unsweetened jams and preserves are naturally sweet and when portions are small, are low in carbohydrates. Other good choices include products sweetened with sucralose. It is always important to pay attention to serving size. A good rule of thumb is that one teaspoon of jam will thinly cover a slice of bread. Also note that packets of sugar substitute each contain about 1 gram of carbohydrate, so if you sweeten six cups of herbal tea in one day, the carbs can add up.

Food Item (Amount)	Carb (g)	Fiber (g)	Net Carbs (g)	Protein (g)	Fat (g)	Cals
Jam/Preserves						
Apple butter (1 tsp)	2.6	0.1	2.5	0.0	0.0	10
Artificially sweetened (1 tsp)	3.6	0.2	3.4	0.0	0.0	1
Grape jelly (1 tsp)	4.7	0.0	4.7	0.0	0.0	20
Jam/preserves (1 tsp)	4.6	0.1	4.5	0.0	0.0	19
Reduced sugar (1 tsp)	3.0	0.2	2.8	0.1	0.1	12
Steele's jams, assorted flavors (1 tbs)	1-2.3	0.0	1-2.3	0.0	0.0	6-10
Syrups						
CHOCOLATE SYRUP						
Hershey's (1 tbs)	11.9	0.5	11.4	0.5	0.2	51
Hershey's Lite (1 tbs)	5.8	0.4	5.4	0.3	0.1	25
Corn Syrup (1 tbs)	15.7	0.0	15.7	0.0	0.0	58
Honey (1 tsp)	5.8	0.0	5.8	0.0	0.0	21
Molasses (1 tsp)	4.4	0.0	4.4	0.0	0.0	17
PANCAKE SYRUP						
Atkins (1 tbs)	0.0	0.0	0.0	0.0	0.0	0
Maple (1 tbs)	13.4	0.0	13.4	0.0	0.0	52
Maple-flavored (1 tbs)	15.1	0.0	15.1	0.0	0.0	57
Reduced calorie (1 tbs)	6.6	0.0	6.6	0.0	0.0	25
Steel's Sugar Free Chocolate Fudge Sauce (1 tbs)	2.5	1.0	1.5	0.5	1.5	23
Sugar						
Brown, packed (1 tsp)	4.5	0.0	4.5	0.0	0.0	17
Maple (1 tsp)	2.7	0.0	2.7	0.0	0.0	11
Powdered, unsifted (1 tsp)	2.5	0.0	2.5	0.0	0.0	10
White (1 tsp)	4.2	0.0	4.2	0.0	0.0	16

Food Item (Amount)	Carb (g)	Fiber (g)	Net Carbs (g)	Protein (g)	Fat (g)	Cals
Sweeteners						
Equal (1 packet)	0.9	0.0	0.9	0.0	0.0	4
Splenda (1 tbs)	1.6	0.0	1.6	0.0	0.0	6
Splendat (1 packe)	1.0	0.0	1.0	0.0	0.0	4
Stevia (1 packet)	1.0	0.0	1.0	0.0	0.0	4
Sugar Twin, brown (1 tsp)	0.4	0.0	0.4	0.0	0.0	1
Sweet'N Low (1 packet)	1.0	0.0	1.0	0.0	0.0	0
Syrup, Atkins, all flavors (1 tbs)	0.0	0	0.0	0.0	0.0	0

SAUCES, GRAVIES AND MARINADES

Reading labels is extremely important in this category. Not only do carb counts vary widely, but many sauces also contain corn syrups and hydrogenated oils, which should be avoided. Be especially careful when buying tomato sauce: Find a brand low in carbs that you like and stock up on it. Marinades are minimally absorbed by the foods they coat, so you may safely halve the total carb count given for marinades. But do avoid slathering barbecue sauce on grilled food—not only will it burn, but more doesn't mean tastier and only adds extra carbs.

Food Item (Amount)	Carb (g)	Fiber (g)	Net Carbs (g)	Protein (g)	Fat (g)	Cals
Sauces						
BARBECUE SAUCE						
Forgione (2 tbs)	1.0	0.0	1.0	0.0	0.0	15
Hunt's Bold Original (1 tbs)	5.4	0.3	5.1	0.2	0.1	23
Kraft Hickory Smoke (1 tbs)	4.5	0.0	4.5	0.0	0.0	20
Kraft Thick 'N Spicy (1 tbs)	6.0	0.0	6.0	0.0	0.0	25
Rocky Mountain Sweetened (2 tbs)	1.0	0.0	1.0	0.0	0.0	15
COCKTAIL SAUCE						
Kraft (2 tbs)	6.5	0.2	6.3	0.5	0.2	30
Steel's Sugar Free (2 tbs)	0.5	0.3	0.3	0.5	0.0	18
Cranberry sauce, whole or jellied (2 tbs)	13.0	0.5	12.5	0.0	0.0	50
PASTA SAUCE						
Contadina Four Cheese (1/4 cup)	6.0	1.0	5.0	1.0	0.5	30
Di Giorno Alfredo (1/4 cup)	2.0	0.0	2.0	4.0	22.0	230
Newman's Own Five Cheese (1/4 cup)	14.0	3.0	11.0	2.0	3.0	90
Newman's Own Sockarooni (1/4 cup)	9.0	3.0	6.0	2.0	2.0	60
Prego Marinara (1/4 cup)	6.0	1.5	4.5	1.0	3.0	55
Prego Traditional (1/4 cup)	10.4	2.0	8.4	1.1	2.5	68
Ragu Old World Style (1/4 cup)	6.1	1.3	4.8	0.9	1.3	40
Rao's (1/4 cup)	2.0	1.0	1.0	2.5	2.0	30
Peanut sauce (2 tbs)	3.6	0.9	2.7	3.9	7.9	94
Pesto sauce (2 tbs)	2.0	0.9	1.2	5.6	14.2	155
SWEET AND SOUR SAUCE						
Kraft (2 tbs)	19.0	16.0	3.0	0.0	0.5	80

Food Item (Amount)	Carb (g)	Fiber (g)	Net Carbs (g)	Protein (g)	Fat (g)	Cals
Steel's Sugar Free (2 tbs)	2.0	0.0	1.0	0.0	0.0	10
TACO SAUCE						
Green (1 tbs)	0.9	0.1	0.8	0.1	0.0	5
Red, Old El Paso, medium (1 tbs)	1.0	0.0	1.0	0.0	0.0	5
Red, Ortega Thick & Smooth (1 tbs)	2.0	0.0	2.0	0.0	0.0	10
Tartar sauce, Kraft (2 tbs)	4.0	0.0	4.0	0.0	10.0	100
TOMATO SAUCE						
Canned (1/4 cup)	4.4	0.9	3.5	0.8	0.1	18
Hunt's Seasoned Tomato Sauce for Pizza (1/4 cup)	5.0	1.0	4.0	1.0	0.0	25
Redpack (1/4 cup)	5.0	1.0	4.0	0.0	0.0	20
Gravy, jarred/canned						
Au jus (2 tbs)	0.8	0.0	0.8	0.4	0.1	5
Beef (2 tbs)	1.4	0.1	1.3	1.1	0.7	15
Chicken (2 tbs)	1.6	0.1	1.5	0.6	1.7	24
Mushroom (2 tbs)	1.6	0.1	1.5	0.4	0.8	15
Turkey (2 tbs)	1.5	0.1	1.4	0.8	0.6	15
Hollandaise sauce (2 tbs)	1.7	0.1	1.6	0.6	2.5	30
Marinades						
A 1 Steak House Classic (1 tbs)	4.0	0.0	4.0	2.0	0.0	15
Annie's Naturals Organic Smoky Campfire (1 tbs)	0.0	0.0	0.0	0.0	3.0	30
Annie's Naturals Organic Spicy Ginger (1 tbs)	2.0	0.0	2.0	0.0	1.0	18
Consorzio California Teriyaki (1 tbs)	5.0	0.0	5.0	1.0	2.0	40
Consorzio Tropical Grill (1 tbs)	3.0	0.0	3.0	0.0	0.0	15

Food Item (Amount)	Carb (g)	Fiber (g)	Net Carbs (g)	Protein (g)	Fat (g)	Cals
KC Masterpiece Hickory & Spice (1 tbs)	7.0	0.0	7.0	0.0	1.5	40
Kikkoman Teriyaki (1 tbs)	2.0	0.0	2.0	1.0	0.0	15
30 Minute Mesquite (1 tbs)	1.0	0.0	1.0	0.0	0.0	5
Salsa						
Desert Pepper 2 Olive Roasted Garlic (2 tbs)	2.0	1.0	1.0	0.0	0.0	10
Doritos Medium (2 tbs)	3.0	1.0	2.0	1.0	0.0	15
Green (2 tbs)	1.0	0.0	1.0	0.0	0.0	10
Newman's Own Roasted Garlic (2 tbs)	2.0	1.0	1.0	1.0	0.0	10
Old El Paso Thick 'N Chunky (2 tbs)	2.0	0.0	2.0	0.0	0.0	10
Red (2 tbs)	2.0	0.5	1.5	0.4	0.1	9

SEASONINGS
AND CONDIMENTS

These products add flavor to most other foods, so keep a variety in your pantry and refrigerator. With the exception of commercial ketchup (which contains corn syrup), most are low in carbs because their intense flavors mean you only need to consume small amounts. A quick tip: To make your own sweet relish, chop up dill pickles, sprinkle with sugar substitute and marinate in the refrigerator for a day.

Food Item (Amount)	Carb (g)	Fiber (g)	Net Carbs (g)	Protein (g)	Fat (g)	Cals
Anchovies, in oil, drained (1)	0.0	0.0	0.0	1.2	0.4	8
Bac'n Pieces, McCormick (1½ tbs)	2.0	0.0	2.0	3.0	1.5	30
Bacon Bits, Oscar Mayer (1 tbs)	0.2	0.0	0.2	2.7	1.3	24
Basil, fresh (1 tbs)	0.1	0.1	0.0	0.1	0.0	1
Basil, ground (1 tsp)	0.9	0.6	0.3	0.2	0.1	4
Capers (1 tbs)	0.4	0.3	0.1	0.2	0.1	2
Caponata (2 tbs)	2.0	2.0	0.0	0.0	2.0	25
Catsup/Ketchup (1 tbs)	4.2	0.2	4.0	0.2	0.1	16
Catsup, Steel's sugar free (1 tbs)	2.0	0.0	2.0	0.0	0.0	10
Chili powder (1 tsp)	1.4	0.9	0.5	0.3	0.4	8
Chives (1 tbs)	0.1	0.1	0.1	0.1	0.0	1
Cilantro, fresh (1 tbs)	0.1	0.1	0.0	0.1	0.0	1
Clam juice (8 fl oz)	0.1	0.0	0.1	0.4	0.0	2
Cumin seed (1 tsp)	0.9	0.2	0.7	0.4	0.5	7
Dill, fresh (1 tbs)	0.0	0.0	0.0	0.0	0.0	0
Fish sauce (1 tsp)	0.2	0.0	0.2	0.3	0.0	2
Garlic, clove (1)	1.0	0.1	0.9	0.2	0.0	4
Ginger root (1 tbs)	0.9	0.1	0.8	0.1	0.0	4
Herbs, dried (oregano, thyme, etc) (1 tsp)	1.0	0.6	0.4	0.2	0.2	5
Hoisin sauce, Steel's (2 tbs)	2.0	1.0	1.0	0.0	0.0	15
Horseradish, prepared (1 tsp)	0.6	0.1	0.4	0.1	0.0	2
Miso paste (1 tbs)	3.0	0.4	2.6	1.9	0.8	27
Mustard, Dijon (1 tsp)	0.6	0.1	0.5	0.3	0.5	
Mustard, yellow (1 tsp)	0.4	0.2	0.2	0.2	0.2	3
Olives, black, large (5)	1.4	0.7	0.7	0.2	2.4	25
Olives, green (5)	0.3	0.2	0.1	0.3	2.5	23
Parsley, fresh (1 tbs)	0.2	0.1	0.1	0.1	0.0	1

Food Item (Amount)	Carb (g)	Fiber (g)	Net Carbs (g)	Protein (g)	Fat (g)	Cals
PEPPERS						
Hot cherry (1)	2.0	1.0	1.0	0.0	0.0	10
Hot red, canned (1)	3.7	1.0	2.8	0.7	0.1	15
Jalapeno, pickled (1)	1.0	0.1	0.8	0.1	0.0	4
Roasted red (1)	1.5	0.0	1.5	0.0	0.0	5
Pickle, dill (1)	2.7	0.8	1.9	0.4	0.1	12
Pickle relish (1 tbs)	5.4	0.2	5.2	0.1	0.1	20
Pickle, sweet (1)	11.1	0.4	10.7	0.1	0.1	41
Sofrito (1 tsp)	0.0	0.0	0.0	0.0	0.0	0
Soy sauce (1 tbs)	1.5	0.0	1.5	0.9	0.0	10
Soy sauce, low sodium (1 tbs)	1.4	0.1	1.2	0.8	0.0	8
Soy sauce, tamari (1 tbs)	1.0	0.2	0.9	1.9	0.0	11
Steak sauce (1 tbs)	2.4	0.3	2.1	0.2	0.0	9
Steak sauce, Newman's Own (1 tbs)	4.0	0.0	4.0	0.0	0.5	20
Sweet and sour sauce, Steel's (1 tbs)	1.0	0.0	1.0	0.0	0.0	5
Tabasco sauce (1 tsp)	0.0	0.0	0.0	0.1	0.0	1
VINEGAR						
Balsamic (1 tbs)	2.3	0.0	2.3	0.0	0.0	10
Cider (1 tbs)	0.9	0.0	0.9	0.0	0.0	2
Red (1 tbs)	1.5	0.0	1.5	0.0	0.0	5
Rice (1 tbs)	0.0	0.0	0.0	0.0	0.0	0
Rice, seasoned (1 tbs)	3.0	0.0	3.0	0.0	0.0	12
White (1 tbs)	0.0	0.0	0.0	0.0	0.0	5
Worcestershire Sauce (1 tsp)	1.0	0.0	1.0	0.0	0.0	4

FATS, OILS AND SALAD DRESSINGS

A good dressing makes the salad and fruity green olive oil will enhance just about any cooked vegetable. Enjoying healthful fats and oils is an important part of doing Atkins and one of its pleasures. When you purchase commercial dressings, be sure to read the ingredient information on the label carefully: While most dressings are relatively low in carbs (except for sweet flavors, such as Honey Dijon), many do contain sugar, hydrogenated oils and artificial flavorings. Your local health food store is a good place to find brands with natural ingredients.

Food Item (Amount)	Carb (g)	Fiber (g)	Net Carbs (g)	Protein (g)	Fat (g)	Cals
Lard (1 tbs)	0.0	0.0	0.0	0.0	12.8	116
Vegetable shortening (Crisco) (1 tbs)	0.0	0.0	0.0	0.0	12.8	113
Oils, Salad and Cooking						
Canola (1 tbs)	0.0	0.0	0.0	0.0	14.0	124
Corn (1 tbs)	0.0	0.0	0.0	0.0	13.6	120
Olive (1 tbs)	0.0	0.0	0.0	0.0	13.5	119
Peanut (1 tbs)	0.0	0.0	0.0	0.0	13.5	119
Safflower (1 tbs)	0.0	0.0	0.0	0.0	13.6	120
Sesame (1 tbs)	0.0	0.0	0.0	0.0	13.6	120
Soybean (1 tbs)	0.0	0.0	0.0	0.0	13.6	120
Salad Dressing						
Annie's Natural Balsamic Vinaigrette (2 tbs)	3.0	0.0	3.0	0.0	10.0	100
Annie's Natural Caesar (2 tbs)	2.0	0.0	2.0	1.0	12.0	120
Kraft Creamy Italian (2 tbs)	3.0	0.0	3.0	0.0	11.0	110
Kraft French (2 tbs)	4.0	0.0	4.0	0.0	12.0	120
Kraft House Italian (2 tbs)	3.0	0.0	3.0	0.0	12.0	120
Kraft Peppercorn Ranch (2 tbs)	1.0	0.0	1.0	1.0	18.0	170
Kraft Thousand Island (2 tbs)	5.0	0.0	5.0	0.0	10.0	110
Marie's Creamy Caesar (2 tbs)	6.0	1.0	5.0	0.5	25.0	250
Marie's Parmesan Ranch (2 tbs)	3.0	0.0	3.0	0.5	19.0	180
Marie's Tangy French (2 tbs)	8.0	0.0	8.0	0.0	11.0	130
Newman's Own Creamy Caesar (2 tbs)	1.0	0.0	1.0	1.0	16.0	150
Newman's Own Parmesan Roasted Garlic (2 tbs)	2.0	0.0	2.0	0.0	11.0	110
Walden Farms Calorie Free (2 tbs)	0.0	0.0	0.0	0.0	0.0	0

Food Item (Amount)	Carb (g)	Fiber (g)	Net Carbs (g)	Protein (g)	Fat (g)	Cals
WishBone Chunky Blue Cheese (2 tbs)	2.0	0.0	2.0	0.5	17.0	170
Wishbone Creamy Roasted Garlic (2 tbs)	3.0	0.0	3.0	0.0	13.0	140
WishBone Deluxe French (2 tbs)	5.0	0.0	5.0	0.0	11.0	120
Wishbone Honey Dijon (2 tbs)	9.0	0.0	9.0	0.5	10.0	130
WishBone Italian (2 tbs)	3.0	0.0	3.0	0.0	9.0	100
WishBone Ranch (2 tbs)	1.0	0.0	1.0	0.0	17.0	160
WishBone Russian (2 tbs)	15.0	0.0	15.0	0.0	6.0	110
WishBone Thousand Island (2 tbs)	7.0	0.0	7.0	0.0	12.0	130
Margarine						
Hard (1 tbs)	0.1	0.0	0.1	0.1	11.4	101
Soft (1 tbs)	0.1	0.0	0.1	0.1	11.4	102
Mayonnaise						
Bestfoods/Hellman's (1 tbs)	0.1	0.0	0.1	0.2	11.2	100
Kraft (1 tbs)	0.0	0.0	0.0	0.0	11.0	100
Light (1 tbs)	1.3	0.0	1.3	0.1	4.9	50
Soybean (1 tbs)	0.4	0.0	0.4	0.2	11.0	99
Miracle Whip (1 tbs)	3.5	0.0	3.5	0.1	4.9	57
Miracle Whip Light (1 tbs)	1.0	0.0	1.0	0.0	5.0	50

SOUPS

The best soups are homemade. They are more flavorful and lower in sodium and carbohydrates—because you control the ingredients. Convenience counts though, and the smartest choices among prepared soups are vegetable soups that are higher in fiber. Since most commercial soups pack at least 15 carb grams —and are only part of a meal—they should be included only when your metabolism allows for greater carbohydrate consumption. A good compromise in terms of convenience and nutritional value is adding fresh chopped cooked or raw veggies to reduced sodium broth. Crumble in a few reduced carb crackers for texture.

Food Item (Amount)	Carb (g)	Fiber (g)	Net Carbs (g)	Protein (g)	Fat (g)	Cals
ALPINE AIR FOODS SOUP IN A CUP						
Bay Shrimp Bisque (1)	6.0	1..0	5.0	6.0	11.0	150
Beefy Vegetable (1)	5.0	1.0	4.0	6.0	3.0	70
Broccoli with Cheddar Cheese (1)	6.0	2.0	4.0	6.0	10.0	140
Chicken with Mushrooms and Roasted Garlic (1)	7.0	1.0	6.0	7.0	8.0	130
Broth/Bouillon, beef (8 oz)	0.1	0.0	0.1	2.6	0.5	16
Broth, cube, all flavors (1)	0.6	0.0	0.6	0.6	0.1	6
CAMPBELL'S, PREPARED FROM CONDENSED						
Bean w/Bacon (8 fl oz)	25.0	7.0	18.0	8.0	5.0	180
Beef Broth (8 fl oz)	1.0	0.0	1.0	3.0	0.0	15
Beef Noodle (8 fl oz)	8.0	1.0	7.0	5.0	2.5	70
Cream of Celery (8 fl oz)	10.0	1.0	9.0	2.0	5.0	90
Chicken broth (8 fl oz)	2.0	0.0	2.0	2.0	2.0	30
Consomme, beef (8 fl oz)	2.0	0.0	2.0	4.0	0.0	25
Cream of Chicken (8 fl oz)	8.0	1.0	7.0	3.0	7.0	110
Chicken Gumbo (8 fl oz)	9.0	1.0	8.0	2.0	1.5	60
Chicken Noodle (8 fl oz)	8.7	0.8	7.9	3.3	1.9	64
Chicken Rice (8 fl oz)	9.0	0.0	9.0	3.0	2.5	70
Clam Chowder, Manhattan (8 fl oz)	12.0	2.0	10.0	2.0	0.5	60
Clam Chowder, New England (8 fl oz)	13.0	1.0	12.0	4.0	2.5	90
Golden Mushroom (8 fl oz)	10.0	1.0	9.0	2.0	3.0	80
Green Pea (8 fl oz)	29.0	5.0	24.0	9.0	3.0	180
Minestrone (8 fl oz)	15.0	4.0	11.0	4.0	1.5	90
Tomato (8 fl oz)	18.0	2.0	16.0	2.0	0.0	80
Turkey Vegetable (8 fl oz)	11.0	2.0	9.0	3.0	2.5	80

Food Item (Amount)	Carb (g)	Fiber (g)	Net Carbs (g)	Protein (g)	Fat (g)	Cals
Vegetable (8 fl oz)	16.0	2.0	14.0	3.0	1.0	90
Vegetable Beef (8 fl oz)	13.0	2.0	11.0	4.0	1.5	80
Vegetarian Vegetable (8 fl oz)	14.0	2.0	12.0	2.0	0.0	60
CAMPBELL'S CHUNKY						
Beef w/Country Vegetables (8 fl oz)	18.0	3.0	15.0	13.0	4.0	160
Classic Chicken Noodle (8 fl oz)	16.0	2.0	14.0	9.0	3.0	130
Minestrone (8 fl oz)	22.0	2.0	20.0	5.0	5.0	140
Vegetable (8 fl oz)	22.0	4.0	18.0	3.0	3.0	130
FANTASTIC SOUP IN A CUP						
Country Lentil (1)	43.0	13.0	30.0	16.0	2.0	250
Creamy Mushroom (1)	24.0	2.0	22.0	6.0	0.0	120
Minestrone (1)	30.0	4.0	26.0	8.0	2.0	170
Split Pea (1)	35.0	8.0	27.0	12.0	1.0	190
HEALTH VALLEY						
Black Bean (1 cup)	25.0	5.0	20.0	7.0	1.0	130
14 Garden Vegetable (1 cup)	17.0	4.0	13.0	6.0	0.0	80
Garden Split Pea with Carrots (1 cup)	20.0	1.0	19.0	5.0	0.0	100
HEALTHY CHOICE						
Hearty Chicken (8 fl oz)	23.0	3.0	20.0	5.0	2.0	130
Chicken w/Rice (8 fl oz)	16.0	3.0	13.0	5.0	2.0	100
New England Clam Chowder (8 fl oz)	24.0	4.0	20.0	5.0	1.5	120
Split Pea w/Ham (8 fl oz)	28.0	5.0	23.0	13.0	2.0	170
Garden Vegetable (8 fl oz)	25.0	3.0	22.0	5.0	0.5	100
KNORR SOUP IN A CUP						
Beef Vegetable Soup(1)	27.0	1.0	26.0	5.0	2.0	150
Red Bean Chili (1)	32.0	8.0	24.0	9.0	1.0	170

Food Item (Amount)	Carb (g)	Fiber (g)	Net Carbs (g)	Protein (g)	Fat (g)	Cals
LIPTON SOUP IN A CUP						
Beefy Mushroom (1)	6.6	0.1	6.5	0.9	0.4	33
Harvest Vegetable (1)	17.0	2.0	15.0	1.0	1.5	90
Vegetable (1)	6.5	1.0	5.5	0.8	0.2	28
NILE SPICE SOUP IN A CUP						
Black Bean (1)	36.0	12.0	24.0	12.0	1.5	170
Cheddar Broccoli (1)	20.0	1.0	19.0	6.0	3.0	130
Chili & Beans (1)	24.7	5.7	19.0	8.2	2.2	151
Tomato & Rice (1)	22.7	1.4	21.3	4.6	2.8	135
PROGRESSO						
Lentil Soup (8 fl oz)	22.0	7.0	15.0	9.0	2.0	140
Escarole In Chicken Broth (8 fl oz)	3.0	1.0	2.0	1.0	1.0	25
Healthy Classics Cream of Broccoli (8 fl oz)	13.3	2.4	10.9	2.4	2.8	88
Healthy Classics Beef Barley (8 fl oz)	20.0	3.1	16.9	11.3	1.9	142
Meatballs & Pasta (8 fl oz)	13.0	0.0	13.0	7.0	7.0	140
Tomato Vegetable (8 fl oz)	15.0	4.0	11.0	3.0	2.0	90
RAMEN IN A CUP						
Fantastic Mandarin Broccoli Big Soup Noodle Bowl (1)	21.0	2.0	19.0	6.0	0.0	110
Nissin Cup Of Noodles Chicken Ramen (1)	36.8	0.0	36.8	5.6	14.1	296

FISH AND SHELLFISH

Most fish and shellfish have no carbohydrates, or very few. The notable exceptions are mussels, oysters and surimi (synthetic crab meat). In addition to being low in carbs, salmon, sardines, mackerel and other fatty fish are good sources of omega-3 fatty acids. The problem with seafood is often the breading. For controlled carb crunchy fish fillets or shrimp, try dredging in equal parts of Atkins™ Bake Mix and finely ground nuts.

Food Item (Amount)	Carb (g)	Fiber (g)	Net Carbs (g)	Protein (g)	Fat (g)	Cals
Fish						
BASS						
Sea Bass, baked (6 oz)	0.0	0.0	0.0	40.2	4.4	211
Striped Bass, baked (6 oz)	0.0	0.0	0.0	38.7	5.1	211
Bluefish, baked (6 oz)	0.0	0.0	0.0	43.7	9.3	270
Catfish, baked (6 oz)	0.0	0.0	0.0	31.8	13.6	259
COD						
Baked (6 oz)	0.0	0.0	0.0	38.8	1.5	179
Dried, salted (3 oz)	0.0	0.0	0.0	53.4	2.0	247
FISH STICKS						
Mrs. Paul's Breaded (6 pieces)	19.0	1.0	18.0	9.0	11.0	210
Mrs. Paul's Crunchy (6 pieces)	21.0	1.0	20.0	10.0	14.0	250
Mrs. Paul's Healthy Treasures (6 pieces)	30.0	3.0	27.0	15.0	4.5	255
Van de Kamp Battered (6 pieces)	18.0	0.0	18.0	11.0	16.0	260
Flounder, baked (6 oz)	0.0	0.0	0.0	41.1	2.6	199
Gefilte, no sugar added (1 piece)	3.0	1.0	2.0	7.0	3.0	80
Gorton's Garlic Butter Grilled Fillets (1 piece)	1.0	0.0	1.0	17.0	3.0	100
HADDOCK						
Baked (6 oz)	0.0	0.0	0.0	40.7	1.6	187
Smoked (6 oz)	0.0	0.0	0.0	42.9	1.6	197
Van de Kamp Battered (2 pieces)	18.0	0.0	18.0	13.0	16.0	260
Halibut, baked (6 oz)	0.0	0.0	0.0	45.4	5.0	238
HERRING						
Vita Herring in Sour Cream (1/4 cup)	8.0	0.0	8.0	7.0	7.0	120

Food Item (Amount)	Carb (g)	Fiber (g)	Net Carbs (g)	Protein (g)	Fat (g)	Cals
Vita Herring Party Snacks (1/4 cup)	10.0	0.0	10.0	9.0	5.0	120
Mackerel, baked (6 oz)	0.0	0.0	0.0	40.6	30.3	446
Mahi-mahi, baked (6 oz)	0.0	0.0	0.0	42.0	1.6	193
Perch, baked (6 oz)	0.0	0.0	0.0	42.3	2.0	199
SALMON						
Baked (6 oz)	0.0	0.0	0.0	37.6	21.0	350
Canned (6 oz)	0.0	0.0	0.0	34.8	12.4	260
Smoked (6 oz)	0.0	0.0	0.0	31.1	7.4	199
SARDINES						
Canned in mustard (6 oz)	0.0	0.0	0.0	27.8	20.4	303
Canned in oil (6 oz)	0.0	0.0	0.0	41.9	19.5	354
Canned in tomato sauce (6 oz)	0.0	0.0	0.0	27.8	20.4	303
Scrod, baked (6 oz)	0.0	0.0	0.0	40.0	1.0	180
Shad, baked (6 oz)	0.0	0.0	0.0	36.9	30.0	429
Snapper, baked (6 oz)	0.0	0.0	0.0	44.7	2.9	218
Swordfish, baked (6 oz)	0.0	0.0	0.0	43.2	8.7	264
Trout, baked (6 oz)	0.0	0.0	0.0	45.3	14.4	323
TUNA						
Baked (6 oz)	0.0	0.0	0.0	50.9	10.7	313
White, canned in oil (6 oz)	0.0	0.0	0.0	45.1	13.7	316
White, canned in water (6 oz)	0.0	0.0	0.0	40.2	5.1	218
Shellfish						
CLAMS						
Canned, drained (6 oz)	8.7	0.0	8.7	43.5	3.3	252
Fried, Gorton's (15 pieces)	20.0	0.0	20.0	8.0	15.0	250
Fried, Mrs. Paul's (6 oz)	58.0	2.0	56.0	16.0	32.0	560

Food Item (Amount)	Carb (g)	Fiber (g)	Net Carbs (g)	Protein (g)	Fat (g)	Cals
CRAB						
Canned, drained (6 oz)	0.0	0.0	0.0	34.9	2.1	168
Steamed (6 oz)	0.0	0.0	0.0	34.4	3.0	174
Surimi (imitation crabmeat) (6 oz)	17.4	0.0	17.4	20.5	2.2	174
Crawfish (6 oz)	0.0	0.0	0.0	32.6	1.9	169
Lobster, steamed (6 oz)	2.2	0.0	2.2	34.9	1.0	167
Mussels, steamed (6 oz)	12.6	0.0	12.6	40.5	7.6	293
OYSTERS						
Canned (6 oz)	6.7	0.0	6.7	12.0	4.2	117
Raw (6 oz)	6.7	0.0	6.7	12.0	4.2	116
Smoked (6 oz)	18.2	12.2	6.1	30.4	18.2	304
Prawns, steamed (6 oz)	0.0	0.0	0.0	35.6	1.8	168
SCALLOPS						
Baked (6 oz)	4.9	0.0	4.9	34.7	6.7	228
Fried, Mrs.Paul's (13 pieces)	27.0	1.0	26.0	12.0	7.0	220
Mrs.Paul's (6 oz)	38.2	1.7	36.5	17.4	13.9	365
SHRIMP						
Cocktail (6 oz)	15.7	3.6	12.0	20.8	1.9	161
Cooked (6 oz)	0.0	0.0	0.0	35.6	1.8	168
Gorton's Popcorn (22 pieces)	28.0	0.0	28.0	10.0	11.0	250
Mrs. Paul's Cajun (21 pieces)	4.0	1.0	3.0	13.0	1.5	90
Van de Kamp Crunchy Butterfly (7 pieces)	30.0	3.0	27.0	10.0	15.0	300
Squid, cooked (6 oz)	6.4	0.0	6.4	32.2	8.0	236

BEEF, PORK AND LAMB

The only higher carbohydrate items in this category are calf's liver and some luncheon meats, such as liverwurst and pastrami. Versatile and readily available, beef, pork and lamb are an important part of a controlled carbohydrate program. This does not mean, however, that portions should be excessively large.

Food Item (Amount)	Carb (g)	Fiber (g)	Net Carbs (g)	Protein (g)	Fat (g)	Cals
Beef and Veal						
BEEF MEALS						
Thomas E. Wilson Seasoned Beef Meatloaf (5 oz)	12.0	1.0	11.0	17.0	16.0	270
Time for Dinner Beef Pot Roast (5 oz)	7.0	0.0	7.0	23.0	5.0	170
BEEF, ROASTED/COOKED						
Brisket (6 oz)	0.0	0.0	0.0	44.0	41.7	563
Chuck (6 oz)	0.0	0.0	0.0	50.1	31.6	498
Chuck eye steak (6 oz)	0.0	0.0	0.0	46.2	41.1	568
Corned beef brisket (6 oz)	0.3	0.0	0.3	33.3	33.8	449
Cubed steak (6 oz)	0.0	0.0	0.0	53.9	8.3	306
Eye round (6 oz)	0.0	0.0	0.0	45.3	24.0	410
Ground chuck (6 oz)	0.0	0.0	0.0	38.9	44.0	562
Ground round (6 oz)	0.0	0.0	0.0	46.7	28.1	454
Jerky (5 oz)	0.0	0.0	0.0	4.0	2.0	35
Prime rib (6 oz)	0.0	0.0	0.0	37.0	56.4	667
Rib eye roast (6 oz)	0.0	0.0	0.0	37.0	56.4	667
Rib eye steak (6 oz)	0.0	0.0	0.0	42.4	37.9	522
Roast (6 oz)	0.0	0.0	0.0	38.7	45.6	576
Roast, deli (6 oz)	2.3	0.0	2.3	34.4	5.2	193
Shell steak (6 oz)	0.0	0.0	0.0	48.7	16.0	352
Short ribs (6 oz)	0.0	0.0	0.0	36.7	71.4	801
Sirloin steak (6 oz)	0.0	0.0	0.0	51.7	13.6	344
Skirt steak (6 oz)	0.0	0.0	0.0	46.2	41.1	568
Tenderloin (6 oz)	0.0	0.0	0.0	40.9	49.2	619
Top loin (6 oz)	0.0	0.0	0.0	51.7	12.3	332
Top sirloin (6 oz)	0.0	0.0	0.0	44.2	30.4	463
Liver, calf (6 oz)	10.4	0.0	10.4	40.5	9.9	304

Food Item (Amount)	Carb (g)	Fiber (g)	Net Carbs (g)	Protein (g)	Fat (g)	Cals
VEAL, ROASTED/COOKED						
Arm shoulder (6 oz)	0.0	0.0	0.0	43.3	14.0	311
Breast (6 oz)	0.0	0.0	0.0	39.6	33.5	472
Cutlet (6 oz)	0.0	0.0	0.0	51.4	29.3	483
Ground (6 oz)	0.0	0.0	0.0	41.5	12.9	293
Loin (6 oz)	0.0	0.0	0.0	51.4	29.3	483
Rib chop (6 oz)	0.0	0.0	0.0	40.8	23.8	388
Round steak (6 oz)	0.0	0.0	0.0	47.6	7.0	265
Scallops (6 oz)	0.0	0.0	0.0	47.8	5.8	255
Shank (6 oz)	0.0	0.0	0.0	43.4	7.9	256
Stew meat (6 oz)	0.0	0.0	0.0	40.2	13.4	292
Lamb and Goat						
Goat, roasted (6 oz)	0.0	0.0	0.0	46.1	5.2	243
LAMB, ROASTED						
Ground (6 oz)	0.0	0.0	0.0	42.1	33.4	481
Leg, bone-in (6 oz)	0.0	0.0	0.0	48.1	13.2	325
Rack, bone-in (6 oz)	0.0	0.0	0.0	44.5	22.6	395
Rib chop (6 oz)	0.0	0.0	0.0	37.6	50.3	614
Shoulder (6 oz)	0.0	0.0	0.0	48.1	13.2	325
Stew meat (6 oz)	0.0	0.0	0.0	57.3	15.0	379
Lunch Meats and Sausage						
Bologna, beef (3 slices)	2.0	0.0	2.0	9.3	24.5	266
Bologna, beef & pork (3 slices)	2.4	0.0	2.4	10.0	24.1	269
Breakfast sausage (1 link)	1.2	0.7	0.5	4.5	1.0	32
Chorizo (2 oz)	1.1	0.0	1.1	13.7	21.7	258
FRANKFURTER						
Beef & pork (2 oz)	1.5	0.0	1.5	6.8	17.0	188
Beef (1)	1.2	0.0	1.2	5.0	13.1	143
Hebrew National (1)	1.0	0.0	1.0	6.0	14.0	150
Ham (6 oz)	1.8	0.0	1.8	28.2	6.6	174
Liverwurst (6 oz)	9.6	3.0	6.6	21.6	43.2	528

Food Item (Amount)	Carb (g)	Fiber (g)	Net Carbs (g)	Protein (g)	Fat (g)	Cals
Olive loaf (3 slices)	7.8	0.0	7.8	10.0	14.0	200
Pastrami, beef (6 oz)	5.2	0.0	5.2	29.3	49.6	594
Pepperoni (5 pieces)	0.8	0.0	0.8	5.8	12.1	137
Pork and beef sausage (1)	0.7	0.0	0.7	3.7	9.8	107
Pork sausage (1)	1.0	0.0	1.0	13.4	17.2	216
Spam (2 oz)	0.8	0.0	0.8	7.4	15.8	174
SALAMI						
Beef (3 pieces)	1.9	0.0	1.9	10.4	14.3	181
Beef and pork (3 pieces)	0.8	0.0	0.8	6.9	10.3	125
Pork (3 pieces)	0.5	0.0	0.5	6.8	10.1	122

Pork

PORK MEALS

Food Item (Amount)	Carb (g)	Fiber (g)	Net Carbs (g)	Protein (g)	Fat (g)	Cals
Hormel Pork Roast Au Jus (5 oz)	0.0	0.0	0.0	29.0	7.0	180
Time for Dinner Pork Loin Roast (5 oz)	3.0	0.0	3.0	27.0	9.0	200
PORK, ROASTED/COOKED						
Bacon (3 pieces)	0.1	0.0	0.1	5.8	9.4	109
Canadian bacon (3 pieces)	0.9	0.0	0.9	16.9	5.9	129
Chop, center cut, bone-in (6 oz)	0.0	0.0	0.0	50.7	14.1	344
Frankfurter (1)	1.5	0.0	1.5	6.4	16.5	181
Ground (6 oz)	0.0	0.0	0.0	43.7	35.3	505
Ham, boneless (6 oz)	0.0	0.0	0.0	38.5	15.3	303
Kielbasa, with beef (2 oz)	0.8	0.0	0.8	7.6	17.2	191
Loin chop, bone-in (6 oz)	0.0	0.0	0.0	37.3	43.3	549
Loin roast (6 oz)	0.0	0.0	0.0	46.1	24.9	422
Pancetta (1 oz)	0.2	0.0	0.2	8.6	14.0	163
Prosciutto (6 oz)	0.9	0.0	0.9	37.4	13.0	281
Sausage, Italian (2 oz)	0.9	0.0	0.9	11.4	14.6	183
Spareribs (6 oz)	0.0	0.0	0.0	49.4	51.5	675
Tenderloin (6 oz)	0.0	0.0	0.0	47.9	8.2	279

POULTRY

Grilled, baked or broiled poultry is virtually carb free. Just be careful with seasonings and cooking methods: Breading, batter, sweet and sour sauces, glazes, barbecue sauces, pastry crusts and sweet dips all sneak in carbs. In general, whether dining out and eating in, the simpler the better.

Food Item (Amount)	Carb (g)	Fiber (g)	Net Carbs (g)	Protein (g)	Fat (g)	Cals
Chicken						
CHICKEN, ROASTED						
Breast filet, skinless (6 oz)	0.0	0.0	0.0	50.7	13.2	335
Breast, with skin, boneless (6 oz)	0.0	0.0	0.0	50.7	13.2	335
Drumstick, skinless, boneless (6 oz)	0.0	0.0	0.0	48.1	9.6	293
Drumstick, with skin (6 oz)	0.0	0.0	0.0	46.0	19.0	367
Ground (6 oz)	0.0	0.0	0.0	49.2	12.6	323
Leg, boneless, with skin (6 oz)	0.0	0.0	0.0	44.2	22.9	395
Light and dark (6 oz)	0.0	0.0	0.0	40.8	22.8	379
Thigh, boneless, with skin (6 oz)	0.0	0.0	0.0	42.6	26.4	420
Wing, boneless (6 oz)	0.0	0.0	0.0	45.7	33.1	493
CHICKEN DISHES, FROZEN						
Banquet Popcorn Chicken (11 pieces)	18.0	1.0	17.0	8.0	8.0	190
Bird's Eye Zesty Garlic Chicken (1 cup)	28.0	1.0	27.0	15.0	11.0	270
Goya Chicken Croquettes (3)	30.0	3.0	27.0	13.0	12.0	280
POT PIES						
Banquet (1)	36.0	1.0	35.0	9.9	22.0	382
Morton (1)	32.0	2.0	30.0	8.0	18.0	320
Pepperidge Farm (1)	40.0	0.0	40.0	12.0	26.0	450
"SKILLET" MEALS						
Bird's Eye Chicken Voila! Pesto Chicken Primavera (1 cup)	24.0	2.0	22.0	15.0	8.0	230
Chicken Helper Four Cheese (1 cup)	27.0	0.0	27.0	24.0	12.0	310

Food Item (Amount)	Carb (g)	Fiber (g)	Net Carbs (g)	Protein (g)	Fat (g)	Cals
Green Giant Chicken Teriyaki Skillet Meal (1½ cups)	45.0	3.0	42.0	15.0	1.5	250
Stouffer's Skillet Sensations Teriyaki Chicken (½ package)	46.0	7.0	39.0	19.0	2.0	280
Uncle Ben's Fiesta Chicken Bowl (1)	55.0	4.0	51.0	22.0	6.0	350
Weaver Chicken Breast Strips (3 each)	13.0	2.0	11.0	14.0	11.0	210
Weaver Original Style Chicken Rondelets (1 each)	10.0	1.0	9.0	10.0	11.0	210
CHICKEN, REFRIGERATED, PREPARED						
Purdue Short Cuts Carved Chicken Breast (½ cup)	1.0	0.0	1.0	19.0	2.0	100
Tyson Roasted Whole Chicken (3 oz)	1.0	0.0	1.0	16.0	11.0	160
Chicken sausage, Aidell's Smoked Chicken & Apple (1 each)	1.0	0.0	1.0	16.0	16.0	210
Cornish hen, roasted (6 oz)	0.0	0.0	0.0	37.9	31.0	442
Duck and Goose						
DUCK, ROASTED						
Breast, without skin (6 oz)	0.0	0.0	0.0	45.0	9.6	279
Whole (6 oz)	0.0	0.0	0.0	26.1	89.2	916
Goose, roasted (6 oz)	0.0	0.0	0.0	42.8	37.3	519
Turkey						
TURKEY, ROASTED						
Breast, without skin (6 oz)	0.0	0.0	0.0	51.1	1.3	230
Ground (6 oz)	0.0	0.0	0.0	46.5	22.4	400
Light and dark (6 oz)	0.1	0.0	0.1	47.6	16.1	349

Food Item (Amount)	Carb (g)	Fiber (g)	Net Carbs (g)	Protein (g)	Fat (g)	Cals
Sausage (2 oz)	0.3	0.0	0.3	9.6	6.4	97
TURKEY POT PIES						
Banquet (1)	38.0	3.0	35.0	10.0	20.0	370
Swanson (1)	42.0	3.0	39.0	10.0	21.0	400
Turkey Jerky, Shelton's (1/2 oz)	1	0	1.0	9	0.5	50

NUTS, NUT BUTTERS AND SEEDS

Nuts and seeds are high in protein, fiber, flavor and fat—which makes a small handful a filling, nutritional and energizing snack. Macadamias, walnuts, pecans and Brazil nuts are top choices because they have a higher fat content and are lower in carbs than other nuts. Add a small amount of chopped nuts for a nice crunch in casseroles and extra flavor in vegetable side dishes. They're also an important ingredient in controlled carb desserts: Finely ground nuts often take the place of white flour.

Food Item (Amount)	Carb (g)	Fiber (g)	Net Carbs (g)	Protein (g)	Fat (g)	Cals
ALMONDS						
Butter (2 tbs)	6.8	1.2	5.6	4.8	18.9	203
Paste (1 oz)	13.6	1.4	12.2	2.6	7.9	130
Slivered, blanched (2 tbs)	3.3	1.6	1.7	3.5	8.6	102
Whole, roasted (24)	5.7	3.4	2.3	6.1	14.6	166
Brazil nuts, roasted (6)	3.6	1.5	2.1	4.1	18.8	186
CASHEWS						
Butter (2 tbs)	8.8	0.6	8.2	5.6	15.8	188
Whole, roasted (2 tbs)	5.6	0.5	5.1	2.6	7.9	98
Chestnuts, roasted (6)	26.7	2.6	24.2	1.6	1.1	124
Coconut, dried, unsweetened (2 tbs)	2.4	1.6	0.8	0.7	6.3	64
Hazelnuts, roasted (2 tbs)	2.8	1.6	1.2	2.5	10.3	106
MACADAMIA NUTS						
Butter (2 tbs)	5.0	0.0	5.0	3.0	24.0	230
Roasted (2 tbs)	2.3	1.4	0.9	1.3	12.7	120
Nutella (2 tbs)	23.0	2.0	21.0	3.0	10.0	200
PEANUTS						
Butter, natural (2 tbs)	6.9	2.1	4.8	7.7	15.9	187
Butter, smooth (2 tbs)	6.2	1.9	4.3	8.1	16.3	190
Oil-roasted (2 tbs)	3.4	1.7	1.8	4.7	8.9	105
Pecans, roasted (2 tbs)	1.9	1.3	0.6	1.2	9.7	93
Pine nuts (2 tbs)	2.4	0.8	1.7	4.1	8.6	96
Pistachios (2 tbs)	4.7	1.6	3.1	3.3	6.9	88
Pumpkin seeds, hulled (2 tbs)	4.3	0.3	4.0	1.5	1.6	36
Sesame seeds (2 tbs)	4.2	2.1	2.1	3.2	8.9	103
Soybeans, roasted (2 tbs)	7.0	1.7	5.3	8.5	4.7	97
Sunflower seeds, hulled (2 tbs)	3.9	1.8	2.1	3.1	8.0	93
Walnuts, halves (2 tbs)	1.7	0.8	0.9	1.9	8.2	82

VEGETABLES

Potatoes are the most popular vegetable in America, but they should be at the bottom of your option list. In terms of nutritional density, dark green vegetables rate number one in antioxidant capacity, and cruciferous vegetables, such as cabbage, broccoli or Brussels sprouts are known to help fight disease. Cooked kale, collards or spinach topped with toasted garlic and olive oil is delicious, as well as among the most healthful foods you can eat. On Lifetime Maintenance, most people can also enjoy moderate portions of higher glycemic veggies such as winter squash, carrots and sweet potatoes, all of which are loaded with beta-carotene.

Food Item (Amount)	Carb (g)	Fiber (g)	Net Carbs (g)	Protein (g)	Fat (g)	Cals
ARTICHOKES						
Whole (1)	13.4	6.5	6.9	4.2	0.2	60
Hearts, frozen (1/2 cup)	7.8	6.0	1.8	2.7	0.4	38
Hearts, marinated (4 pieces)	4.0	2.0	2.0	0.0	4.0	40
ASPARAGUS						
Steamed (4 spears)	2.5	1.0	1.6	1.6	0.2	14
Canned (4 pieces)	1.8	1.2	0.6	1.5	0.5	14
Frozen, steamed (1/2 cup)	4.4	1.4	2.9	2.7	0.4	25
Bamboo shoots, canned, sliced (1/2 cup)	2.1	0.9	1.2	1.1	0.3	12
BEANS						
Green, steamed (1/2 cup)	4.9	2.0	2.9	1.2	0.2	22
Green Giant Green Bean Casserole (2/3 cup)	9.0	2.0	7.0	2.0	5.0	90
Yellow wax, steamed (1/2 cup)	4.9	2.1	2.9	1.2	0.2	22
Beets, canned (1/2 cup)	6.1	1.4	4.7	0.8	0.1	26
Bok choi (1/2 cup)	1.5	1.4	0.2	1.3	0.1	10
Broccoflower, steamed (1/2 cup)	4.8	2.5	2.3	2.3	0.2	25
BROCCOLI						
Flowerets, raw (1/2 cup)	1.9	1.1	0.8	1.1	0.1	10
Frozen, chopped, steamed (1/2 cup)	4.9	2.8	2.2	2.9	0.1	26
BROCCOLI DISHES						
Bird's Eye Broccoli w/Cheese Sauce (1/2 cup)	7.1	1.9	5.2	4.3	3.2	70
Green Giant Broccoli & Three Cheese Sauce (1/2 cup)	5.0	2.0	3.0	3.0	2.5	50
Broccoli Rabe, raw (1/2 cup)	2.0	0.0	2.0	1.3	0.0	10
Broccolini, steamed (1/2 cup)	8.0	1.3	6.7	4.0	0.0	47

Food Item (Amount)	Carb (g)	Fiber (g)	Net Carbs (g)	Protein (g)	Fat (g)	Cals
Brussels sprouts, steamed (1/2 cup)	6.8	2.0	4.7	2.0	0.4	30
CABBAGE						
Chinese (1/2 cup)	1.4	1.4	0.0	0.9	0.1	8
Green, shredded, raw (1/2 cup)	1.9	0.8	1.1	0.5	0.1	9
Green, steamed (1/2 cup)	3.3	1.7	1.6	0.8	0.3	17
Red, shredded, raw (1/2 cup)	2.1	0.7	1.4	0.5	0.1	9
Savoy, steamed (1/2 cup)	3.9	2.0	1.9	1.3	0.1	17
Cardoon, steamed (1/2 cup)	3.9	1.2	2.7	0.6	0.1	16
CARROT						
Sliced, steamed (1/2 cup)	8.2	2.6	5.6	0.9	0.1	35
Whole, 7 1/2" long, raw (1)	7.3	2.2	5.1	0.7	0.1	31
Cassava/Yuca, cooked (1/2 cup)	26.3	1.3	25.1	0.9	0.2	111
CAULIFLOWER						
Raw (1/2 cup)	2.6	1.3	1.4	1.0	0.1	13
Steamed (1/2 cup)	2.6	1.7	0.9	1.1	0.3	14
CAULIFLOWER DISHES						
Bird's Eye Cauliflower w/ Cheese Sauce (1/2 cup)	6.8	1.8	5.0	3.8	2.9	64
Green Giant Cauliflower & Cheese Flavored Sauce (1/2 cup)	7.0	1.0	6.0	2.0	2.5	60
CELERY						
Steamed (1/2 cup)	3.0	1.2	1.8	0.6	0.1	14
Raw, (1 stalk)	1.5	0.7	0.8	0.3	0.1	6
Celeriac, cooked (1/2 cup)	4.6	0.9	3.6	0.7	0.2	21
Chard, steamed (1/2 cup)	3.6	1.8	1.8	1.7	0.1	18
Chayote, steamed (1/2 cup)	4.1	2.2	1.8	0.5	0.4	19
Coleslaw, with dressing (1/2 cup)	7.5	0.9	6.6	0.8	1.6	41

Food Item (Amount)	Carb (g)	Fiber (g)	Net Carbs (g)	Protein (g)	Fat (g)	Cals
Collards, steamed (1/2 cup)	4.7	2.7	2.0	2.0	0.3	25
CORN						
Canned (1/2 cup)	15.2	1.6	13.6	2.2	0.8	66
Cob (1)	19.3	2.2	17.2	2.6	1.0	83
Cream style, canned (1/2 cup)	23.2	1.5	21.7	2.2	0.5	92
Kernels (1/2 cup)	14.7	2.1	12.6	2.5	0.9	66
Cucumber slices (1/2 cup)	1.4	0.4	1.0	0.4	0.1	7
Dandelion greens (1/2 cup)	3.4	1.5	1.8	1.1	0.3	17
Eggplant, broiled (1/2 cup)	3.3	1.2	2.1	0.4	0.1	14
Endive (1/2 cup)	1.8	1.4	0.4	0.4	0.1	8
Fava beans, steamed (1/2 cup)	16.7	4.6	12.1	6.5	0.3	94
FENNEL						
Braised (1/2 cup)	2.8	1.3	1.5	0.6	0.1	12
Raw (1/2 cup)	3.2	1.4	1.8	0.5	0.1	13
Garlic cloves (1)	1.0	0.1	0.9	0.2	0.0	4
Jerusalem artichoke, raw (1/2 cup)	13.1	1.2	11.9	1.5	0.0	57
Jicama, raw (1/2 cup)	5.7	3.2	2.5	0.5	0.1	25
Kale, steamed (1/2 cup)	3.4	1.3	2.1	1.9	0.3	20
Kohlrabi, steamed (1/2 cup)	5.5	0.9	4.6	1.5	0.1	24
LETTUCE						
Boston/Bibb (1/2 cup)	0.7	0.3	0.4	0.4	0.1	4
Iceberg (1/2 cup)	0.6	0.4	0.2	0.3	0.1	3
Looseleaf/mesclun (1/2 cup)	1.0	0.5	0.5	0.4	0.1	5
Romaine (1/2 cup)	0.7	0.5	0.2	0.5	0.1	4
MIXED VEGETABLES, FROZEN						
BIRD'S EYE						
Asparagus Stir Fry (1 cup)	8.0	1.5	16.5	2.5	0.3	45

Food Item (Amount)	Carb (g)	Fiber (g)	Net Carbs (g)	Protein (g)	Fat (g)	Cals
California Style Vegetables (1/2 cup)	9.0	3.0	6.0	3.0	5.0	100
Pepper Stir-Fry (1 cup)	5.0	1.0	4.0	1.0	0.0	25
Rotetti Pasta & Vegetables (1/2 cup)	5.5	1.0	4.5	5.0	4.0	95
GREEN GIANT						
Mixed Vegetables (3/4 cup)	10.0	2.0	8.0	2.0	0.0	50
Teriyaki Vegetables (1 1/4 cups)	6.0	2.0	4.0	2.0	5.0	80
MUSHROOMS						
Portabello (4 oz)	5.8	1.7	4.1	2.8	0.2	29
Shiitake, cooked (1/2 cup)	10.4	1.5	8.8	1.1	0.2	40
Straw, canned (1/2 cup)	4.2	2.3	2.0	3.5	0.6	29
Whole, raw (1/2 cup)	2.0	0.6	1.4	1.4	0.2	12
Mustard greens, steamed (1/2 cup)	1.5	1.4	0.1	1.6	0.2	11
Nopales (cactus pads), cooked (1/2 cup)	2.4	1.5	1.0	1.0	0.0	11
Okra, steamed (1/2 cup)	5.8	2.0	3.8	1.5	0.1	26
Onions, chopped, raw (1/2 cup)	6.9	1.4	5.5	0.9	0.1	30
Parsley, chopped (1 tbs)	0.2	0.1	0.1	0.1	0.0	1
Parsnips, steamed (1/2 cup)	15.2	3.1	12.1	1.0	0.2	63
Pea pods/Snow peas (1/2 cup)	5.6	2.2	3.4	2.6	0.2	34
Peas, frozen (1/2 cup)	9.9	3.4	6.5	3.8	0.3	55
PEPPERS						
Green, raw (1/2 cup)	4.8	1.3	3.5	0.7	0.1	20
Red, raw (1/2 cup)	4.8	1.5	3.3	0.7	0.1	20
POTATO						
Au Gratin, Betty Crocker (1/2 cup)	23.0	1.0	22.0	3.0	6.0	150
Baked, small (1/2)	11.6	1.1	10.5	1.1	0.1	50

Food Item (Amount)	Carb (g)	Fiber (g)	Net Carbs (g)	Protein (g)	Fat (g)	Cals
Boiled (1/2 cup)	15.6	1.4	14.2	1.3	0.1	67
French fries, frozen (10)	15.8	2.0	13.9	1.6	3.8	101
Hash browns, frozen, cooked (1/2 cup)	21.9	1.6	20.4	2.5	9.0	170
Hash Browns, Toaster, Oreida (2 patties)	25.0	2.0	23.0	2.0	12.0	220
Idahoan Real Potato Hashbrowns (1/2 cup)	14.3	1.6	12.8	1.3	3.7	95
Mashed, Boston Market (1/2 cup)	23.0	1.0	22.0	3.0	9.0	180
Mashed, from flakes, prepared (1/2 cup)	15.8	2.4	13.4	2.0	5.9	119
Scalloped, Betty Crocker (1/2 cup)	23.0	1.0	22.0	3.0	6.0	150
PUMPKIN						
Boiled (1/2 cup)	6.0	1.4	4.6	0.9	0.1	25
Canned (1/2 cup)	9.2	5.1	4.1	2.1	0.0	41
Radicchio (1/2 cup)	0.9	0.2	0.7	0.3	0.1	5
Radishes (10)	1.6	0.7	0.9	0.3	0.2	9
Rutabaga, boiled (1/2 cup)	7.4	1.5	5.9	1.1	0.2	33
Sauerkraut (1/2 cup)	5.1	3.0	2.1	1.1	0.2	22
Scallions/green onions (1/2 cup)	3.7	1.3	2.4	0.9	0.1	16
Shallots (1/2 cup)	13.4	0.6	12.9	2.0	0.1	58
Sorrel, cooked (1/2 cup)	1.5	1.3	0.2	0.9	0.3	10
SPINACH						
Creamed, Bird's Eye (1/2 cup)	7.0	1.0	6.0	3.0	7.0	100
Creamed, Green Giant (1/2 cup)	10.0	2.0	8.0	4.0	3.0	80
Frozen, steamed (1/2 cup)	5.1	2.9	2.2	3.0	0.2	27
Raw (1/2 cup)	0.5	0.4	0.1	0.4	0.1	3

Food Item (Amount)	Carb (g)	Fiber (g)	Net Carbs (g)	Protein (g)	Fat (g)	Cals
SPROUTS, RAW						
Alfalfa (1/2 cup)	0.6	0.4	0.2	0.7	0.1	5
Bean (1/2 cup)	3.1	1.0	2.1	1.6	0.0	16
SQUASH						
Acorn, baked (1/2 cup)	14.9	4.5	10.4	1.2	0.1	57
Acorn, boiled (1/2 cup)	10.8	3.2	7.6	0.8	0.1	42
Butternut, baked, cubes (1/2 cup)	10.8	2.9	7.9	0.9	0.1	41
Butternut, baked, mashed (1/2 cup)	12.9	3.4	9.4	1.1	0.1	49
Hubbard, boiled, mashed (1/2 cup)	7.6	3.4	4.2	1.8	0.4	35
Spaghetti, cooked (1/2 cup)	5.0	1.1	3.9	0.5	0.2	21
Summer/Yellow, raw (1/2 cup)	2.5	1.1	1.4	0.7	0.1	11
Summer/Yellow, steamed (1/2 cup)	3.9	1.3	2.6	0.8	0.3	18
Zucchini, raw (1/2 cup)	1.9	0.8	1.1	0.8	0.1	9
Zucchini, steamed (1/2 cup)	2.6	1.1	1.5	1.1	0.1	13
SWEET POTATO						
Baked, medium (1/2)	13.8	1.7	12.1	1.0	0.1	59
Boiled (1/2)	18.3	1.4	17.0	1.3	0.2	79
Candied (1/2 cup)	27.3	2.4	25.0	0.9	3.2	134
Mashed (1/2 cup)	39.8	3.0	36.9	2.7	0.5	172
Tomatillo, chopped (1/2 cup)	3.9	1.3	2.6	0.6	0.7	21
TOMATO						
Cherry (10)	7.9	1.9	6.0	1.4	0.6	36
Plum (1)	2.9	0.7	2.2	0.5	0.2	13
Small (1 each, 3 oz)	4.2	1.0	3.2	0.8	0.3	19
Sun-dried, in oil (2 tbs)	3.2	0.8	2.4	0.7	1.9	29

Food Item (Amount)	Carb (g)	Fiber (g)	Net Carbs (g)	Protein (g)	Fat (g)	Cals
TOMATO PRODUCTS, CANNED						
Diced, in juice (1/4 cup)	2.5	0.5	2.0	0.5	0.0	13
Paste (2 tbs)	6.3	1.3	5.0	1.2	0.2	27
Pomi (1/2 cup)	5.0	3.0	2.0	1.0	0.0	30
Puree (2 tbs)	3.0	0.6	2.4	0.5	0.1	13
Recipe Ready Diced, Contadina (1/2 cup)	10.0	1.0	9.0	1.0	0.0	45
Sauce, Del Monte (1/4 cup)	4.0	0.5	3.5	1.0	0.0	20
Sauce, Contadina (1/4 cup)	3.0	0.5	2.5	1.0	0.0	15
Stewed, Contadina (1/2 cup)	9.0	1.0	8.0	1.0	0.0	35
Taro, cooked (1/2 cup)	4.7	0.7	4.0	2.9	0.5	30
TURNIP GREENS						
Frozen, chopped (1/2 cup)	3.0	2.1	1.0	2.0	0.3	18
Raw, steamed (1/2 cup)	3.1	2.5	0.6	0.8	0.2	14
TURNIPS						
Boiled, cubes (1/2 cup)	3.8	1.6	2.3	0.6	0.1	16
Boiled, mashed (1/2 cup)	5.6	2.3	3.3	0.8	0.1	24
Waterchestnuts (1/2 cup)	8.7	1.8	7.0	0.6	0.0	35
Watercress (1/2 cup)	0.2	0.2	0.0	0.4	0.0	2
Yams, canned, mashed (1/2 cup)	29.7	2.2	27.5	2.5	0.3	129
Yuca, raw (1/2 cup)	39.2	1.9	37.3	1.4	0.3	165

GRAINS, PASTA AND RICE

Bland, chewy and comforting, grains, pasta and rice are permitted in moderation once you're close to your goal weight. Whole grain varieties, which are high in fiber, are preferable nutritionally to processed grains (i.e., brown rice instead of white rice). Some grains, such as buckwheat, bulgur and wheat germ are high in protein. Look for controlled carb pastas and other grain dishes

Food Item (Amount)	Carb (g)	Fiber (g)	Net Carbs (g)	Protein (g)	Fat (g)	Cals
Grains						
Barley, cooked (1/2 cup)	22.2	3.0	19.2	1.8	0.4	97
BRAN						
Oat (2 tbs)	7.8	1.8	6.0	2.0	0.8	29
Wheat (2 tbs)	4.7	3.1	1.6	1.1	0.3	16
Bulgur, cooked (1/2 cup)	16.9	4.1	12.8	2.8	0.2	76
Cornmeal (2 tbs)	13.4	1.3	12.1	1.5	0.3	63
Hominy, cooked (1/2 cup)	11.8	2.1	9.7	1.2	0.7	59
Kasha (buckwheat groats), cooked (1/2 cup)	74.3	9.4	64.8	11.6	2.7	343
Masa (corn flour) (2 tbs)	10.9	1.4	9.5	1.3	0.5	52
Millet, cooked (1/2 cup)	28.4	1.6	26.8	4.2	1.2	143
Quinoa, dry (1/4 cup)	29.3	2.5	26.8	5.6	2.5	159
Tabbouleh, dry (1/4 cup)	26.0	6.0	20.0	4.0	0.5	120
Wheat Germ-Toasted (2 tbs)	7.0	1.8	5.2	4.1	1.5	54
Pasta and Couscous						
COUSCOUS						
Couscous, cooked (1/2 cup)	18.2	1.1	17.1	3.0	0.1	88
Casbah Sahara Cheddar Broccoli (1/2 cup)	9.8	0.3	9.6	2.2	1.1	55
Fantastic, w/Lentils, Meal in a Cup (1)	47.0	9.0	38.0	12.0	1.0	220
Near East Couscous Broccoli & Cheese (1/2 cup)	21.0	1.5	19.5	4.0	2.5	120
MACARONI AND CHEESE						
Amy's, frozen (1/2 cup)	20.5	1.5	19.0	7.0	7.0	180
Kraft, prepared (1/2 cup)	22.0	0.5	21.5	7.0	5.0	160
Morton, frozen (1/2 cup)	17.0	1.5	15.5	4.5	4.0	120

Food Item (Amount)	Carb (g)	Fiber (g)	Net Carbs (g)	Protein (g)	Fat (g)	Cals
NOODLES, COOKED						
Egg (1/2 cup)	19.9	0.9	19.0	3.8	1.2	106
Japanese somen (1/2 cup)	24.2	1.4	22.8	3.5	0.2	115
Rice (1/2 cup)	21.9	0.9	21.0	0.8	0.2	96
Thai rice (1/2 cup)	24.5	1.0	23.5	1.5	0.1	105
Udon (brown rice), dry (1 oz)	19.6	1.6	18.0	4.1	1.0	103
PASTA, COOKED						
Fresh (4 oz)	28.3	2.0	26.3	5.8	1.2	149
Low carb, Atkins, dry (3/4 cup)	10.0	7.0	3.0	28.0	1.0	160
Macaroni, protein-enriched (1/2 cup)	17.8	0.9	16.9	5.1	0.1	94
Plain, all shapes (1/2 cup)	19.8	0.9	18.9	3.3	0.5	99
Ravioli, Celetano, frozen (4)	40.0	2.0	38.0	12.0	6.0	260
Spinach (1/2 cup)	18.3	2.5	15.9	3.2	0.4	91
Whole wheat (1/2 cup)	18.6	2.0	16.6	3.7	0.4	87
PASTA, SPECIALTY, COOKED						
Corn (1/2 cup)	22.5	3.1	19.4	2.1	0.6	101
Quinoa (1/2 cup)	17.5	1.2	16.3	2.0	1.0	90
Rice (1/2 cup)	23.5	1.5	22.0	1.0	0.0	92
Semolina (1/2 cup)	20.6	1.0	19.7	3.8	0.7	102
Sesame rice (1/2 cup)	18.5	2.0	16.5	4.0	1.0	100
Spelt (1/2 cup)	20.0	2.5	17.5	4.0	0.8	95
PASTA DISHES						
Angel Hair Pasta with Herbs, Pasta Roni (1 cup)	42.0	2.0	40.0	9.0	13.0	320
Lasagne with Sauce, Celentano, frozen (7 oz)	29.0	2.0	27.0	11.0	12.0	270
Noodles & Sauce, Beef Flavor, Lipton (1 cup)	42.0	2.0	40.0	8.0	10.0	280

Food Item (Amount)	Carb (g)	Fiber (g)	Net Carbs (g)	Protein (g)	Fat (g)	Cals
Penne with Tomato Mushroom Sauce, Classico (1 container)	98.0	12.0	86.0	15.0	6.0	510
Ravioli, beef in tomato and meat sauce, canned (1 cup)	36.9	3.7	33.2	8.4	5.4	229
Spaghetti, w/tomato sauce & cheese, canned (1/2 cup)	19.3	1.3	18.0	2.8	0.8	95

Rice

RICE, COOKED

Food Item (Amount)	Carb (g)	Fiber (g)	Net Carbs (g)	Protein (g)	Fat (g)	Cals
Basmati, dry (1/4 cup)	39.2	1.1	38.0	4.0	0.7	179
Brown (1/2 cup)	22.4	1.8	20.6	2.5	0.9	108
Short grain risotto (1/2 cup)	26.7	0.9	25.8	2.2	0.2	121
White (1/2 cup)	22.3	0.3	21.9	2.1	0.2	103
Wild (1/2 cup)	17.5	1.5	16.0	3.3	0.3	83

RICE AND GRAIN DISHES

Food Item (Amount)	Carb (g)	Fiber (g)	Net Carbs (g)	Protein (g)	Fat (g)	Cals
Casbah Spanish Pilaf, cooked (1/2 cup)	24.0	0.7	23.3	2.7	0.3	107
Lipton Rice & Sauce, Chicken Flavor, dry (1/4 cup)	24.0	0.5	23.5	3.5	1.0	120
Lipton Rice & Sauce, Chicken Risotto, dry (1/4 cup)	22.0	0.5	21.5	3.5	1.0	115
Near East Brown Rice Pilaf, cooked (1/2 cup)	20.0	1.5	18.5	2.5	2.2	105
Near East Wheat Pilaf, cooked (1/2 cup)	21.0	2.5	18.5	3.0	1.8	105

BEANS, LEGUMES AND TOFU

Tofu is permitted in Induction, but you should not add beans and legumes back in to your diet until you are well into OWL or even in the Pre-Maintenance phase. High in fiber, protein and a variety of minerals and vitamins, beans and other legumes are composed of carbohydrates with a fairly low glycemic index (although they vary from type to type). This means that that they are digested relatively slowly, making you feel fuller longer. And unlike carbs with a higher glycemic index, which raise your blood-sugar level quickly, beans and other legumes are slowly absorbed in the bloodstream. Tofu and other soy products are known to help lower cholesterol and, in moderation, can be helpful for women in menopause. On a culinary note, beans, legumes and especially tofu are bland, so spice them up!

Food Item (Amount)	Carb (g)	Fiber (g)	Net Carbs (g)	Protein (g)	Fat (g)	Cals
Beans and Legumes						
BAKED BEANS						
with pork (1/2 cup)	25.3	7....0	18.3	6.6	2.0	134
Vegetarian (1/2 cup)	26.1	6.4	19.7	6.1	0.6	118
BEAN DIP						
Regular (2 tbs)	6.0	0.0	6.0	2.0	1.0	40
Black Bean (2 tbs)	5.0	1.0	4.0	1.0	0.0	25
Beans w/pork & tomato sauce, canned (1/2 cup)	24.5	6.1	18.5	6.5	1.3	124
Black Beans (1/2 cup)	20.4	7.5	12.9	7.6	0.5	114
Black-eyed peas (1/2 cup)	17.9	5.6	12.3	6.7	0.5	100
Chickpeas/Garbanzo Beans (1/2 cup)	20.0	7.0	13.0	5.0	2.5	120
CHILI, CANNED						
Con carne w/beans (1/2 cup)	14.1	4.7	9.4	11.6	4.7	147
Vegetarian w/beans (1/2 cup)	19.0	4.9	14.1	6.0	0.4	103
Falafel (2-oz patty)	18.1	3.2	14.9	7.6	10.1	189
Great northern beans (1/2 cup)	18.7	6.2	12.5	7.4	0.4	104
Hummus (2 tbs)	6.2	1.6	4.6	1.5	2.6	53
Kidney beans (1/2 cup)	19.8	8.2	11.6	8.1	0.1	110
Lentils (1/2 cup)	19.9	7.8	12.1	8.9	0.4	115
Lima beans, baby (1/2 cup)	21.2	7.0	14.2	7.3	0.4	115
Navy beans (1/2 cup)	23.9	5.8	18.1	7.9	0.5	129
Peas, split (1/2 cup)	20.7	8.1	12.6	8.2	0.4	116
Pink beans (1/2 cup)	23.6	4.5	19.1	7.7	0.4	126
Pinto beans (1/2 cup)	21.9	7.4	14.6	7.0	0.4	117
Refried beans, canned (1/2 cup)	19.6	6.7	12.9	6.9	1.6	118
Soybeans, green (1/2 cup)	10.0	3.8	6.2	11.1	5.8	127

Food Item (Amount)	Carb (g)	Fiber (g)	Net Carbs (g)	Protein (g)	Fat (g)	Cals
Tofu						
Firm (1/2 cup)	5.4	2.9	2.5	19.9	11.0	183
Regular (1/2 cup)	2.3	0.4	2.0	10.0	5.9	94
Silken, firm (1/2 cup)	2.7	0.1	2.6	7.8	3.1	70
Silken, soft (1/2 cup)	3.2	0.1	3.1	5.4	3.1	62

DESSERTS

Products especially made for individuals following a controlled carb program are your best bet here. In second place are sugar-free desserts (though many contain milk, which is high in carbs). Even when desserts are low in carbohydrates it's important to keep in mind that you need not eat one at the end of every meal. Set a weekly limit for yourself and stick to it. In nutritional terms, a cup of fresh berries with a dollop of whipped cream is always your best choice.

Food Item (Amount)	Carb (g)	Fiber (g)	Net Carbs (g)	Protein (g)	Fat (g)	Cals
Frozen Yogurt						
BEN & JERRY'S						
Cherry Garcia (1/2 cup)	31.0	0.0	31.0	4.0	3.0	170
Chocolate Fudge Brownie (1/2 cup)	36.0	1.0	35.0	6.0	3.0	190
EDY'S/DREYERS						
Heath Toffee Crunch (1/2 cup)	18.0	0.0	18.0	2.0	4.0	120
Vanilla (1/2 cup)	17.0	0.0	17.0	2.0	2.5	100
HÄAGEN-DAZS						
Chocolate (1/2 cup)	28.0	0.8	27.3	6.0	0.0	140
Vanilla (1/2 cup)	29.0	0.0	29.0	6.0	0.0	140
Gelatin						
Gelatin dessert, prepared (1/2 cup)	18.9	0.0	18.9	1.6	0.0	80
HandiSnacks Gel Snacks (1)	20.0	0.0	20.0	0.0	0.0	80
Sugar-Free Jell-O Gelatin Snacks (1)	0.0	0.0	0.0	1.3	0.0	7
Sugar free gelatin (1/2 cup)	0.8	0.0	0.8	1.3	0.0	8
Ice Cream						
BEN & JERRY'S						
Cherry Garcia (1/2 cup)	25.0	0.0	25.0	4.0	16.0	240
Chocolate Chip Cookie Dough (1/2 cup)	30.0	0.0	30.0	4.0	17.0	270
Chocolate Fudge Brownie (1/2 cup)	33.0	2.0	31.0	4.0	14.0	250
NY Fudge Crunch (1/2 cup)	28.0	2.0	26.0	5.0	20.0	290
BREYERS						
Butter Pecan (1/2 cup)	14.0	0.0	14.0	3.0	12.0	170

Food Item (Amount)	Carb (g)	Fiber (g)	Net Carbs (g)	Protein (g)	Fat (g)	Cals
Chocolate (1/2 cup)	18.0	1.0	17.0	2.0	9.0	160
French Vanilla (1/2 cup)	14.0	0.0	14.0	3.0	10.0	160
Vanilla (1/2 cup)	15.0	0.0	15.0	3.0	9.0	150
HAAGEN-DAZS						
Chocolate (1/2 cup)	22.0	1.0	21.0	5.0	18.0	270
Coffee (1/2 cup)	21.0	0.0	21.0	5.0	18.0	270
Rum Raisin (1/2 cup)	22.0	0.0	22.0	4.0	17.0	270
Strawberry (1/2 cup)	23.0	0.8	22.3	4.0	16.0	250
STARBUCKS						
Classic Coffee (1/2 cup)	26.0	0.0	26.0	5.0	12.0	230
Java Chip (1/2 cup)	29.0	0.0	29.0	4.0	13.0	250
Mousse						
Expert Food Mousse Mix (1 tsp)	4.0	4.0	0.0	2.0	0.0	24
From instant (1/2 cup)	23.0	0.0	23.0	5.0	9.0	190
Non-Dairy						
Rice Dream Vanilla Non-Dairy Dessert (1/2 cup)	23.0	1.0	22.0	0.0	6.0	150
Sherbet, various flavors (1/2 cup)	30.1	0.0	30.1	1.1	2.0	137
Soy Delicious Creamy Fudge Bar (1)	25.0	2.0	23.0	3.0	4.0	140
Tofutti Life Lite Tofutti, various flavors (1/2 cup)	21.0	0.0	21.0	2.0	11.0	200
Tofutti Life Lite Chocolate Cutie (1)	21.0	0.0	21.0	2.0	5.0	140
Miscellaneous Frozen Treats						
Dove Miniatures (1)	6.0	0.0	6.0	1.0	4.0	60
Edy's Whole Fruit Fruit Bar (1)	13.0	0.0	13.0	0.0	0.0	60
Frozen fruit bar, most flavors (3 oz)	18.6	0.0	18.6	1.1	0.0	75
Frozen fruit bar with cream (2 oz)	19.3	0.1	19.2	1.0	1.3	86

Food Item (Amount)	Carb (g)	Fiber (g)	Net Carbs (g)	Protein (g)	Fat (g)	Cals
Fudgsicle, No Sugar Added (1)	9.0	1.0	8.0	1.0	0.5	45
Klondike No Sugar Added Bar (1)	19.0	1.0	18.0	4.0	10.0	190
Nestle Crunch No Sugar Added Vanilla Bar (1)	16.0	0.0	16.0	1.0	8.0	140
Nestle Icescreamers NesQuik Pop (1)	14.0	2.0	12.0	1.0	4.5	100
Ocean Spray No Sugar Added Fruit Juice Bar (1)	6.0	0.0	6.0	0.0	0.0	25
Popsicle (1)	11.0	0.0	11.0	0.0	0.0	45
Popsicle, Sugar Free (1)	3.0	0.0	3.0	0.0	0.0	15
Starbucks Mocha Frappuccino Bar (1)	22.0	3.0	19.0	4.0	2.0	120
Yoplait Double Fruit Smoothies (1)	11.0	0.0	11.0	1.0	0.0	45
Pudding						
Banana, made with whole milk (1/2 cup)	28.8	0.0	28.8	4.0	4.3	166
Chocolate, made with whole milk (1/2 cup)	27.6	1.5	26.2	4.6	4.6	163
Egg custard, made with whole milk (1/2 cup)	23.4	0.0	23.4	5.5	5.5	162
Rice, made with 2% milk (1/2 cup)	30.0	0.0	30.0	5.0	2.5	160
Tapioca, made with whole milk (1/2 cup)	27.6	0.0	27.6	4.1	4.1	161
Vanilla, made with whole milk (1/2 cup)	28.0	0.0	28.0	3.8	4.1	162

Food Item (Amount)	Carb (g)	Fiber (g)	Net Carbs (g)	Protein (g)	Fat (g)	Cals
READY-MADE PUDDING						
Jell-O Chocolate (1)	28.0	0.0	28.0	3.0	5.0	160
Jell-O Vanilla (1)	25.0	0.0	25.0	3.0	5.0	160
Kozy Shack Rice (1/2 cup)	22.0	0.0	22.0	4.0	3.0	130
Swiss Miss Chocolate Vanilla Swirl (1)	26.0	0.0	26.0	2.0	6.0	160
Swiss Miss Lemon Meringue Pie (1)	30.0	0.0	30.0	0.0	3.0	150
Sorbet						
Häagen-Dazs Chocolate (1/2 cup)	28.0	2.0	26.0	2.0	0.0	120
Häagen-Dazs Raspberry (1/2 cup)	30.0	2.0	28.0	0.0	0.0	120
Häagen-Dazs Zesty Lemon (1/2 cup)	31.0	0.5	30.5	0.0	0.0	120
Whipped Topping						
Cool Whip Lite (2 tbs)	3.0	0.0	0.0	0.0	1.0	20
Cool Whip Regular (2 tbs)	3.0	0.0	0.0	0.0	1.5	25

CAKES, PIES AND BROWNIES

Occasionally, on Lifetime Maintenance, you might splurge on a small slice of pie or piece of cake. When you do so, make sure that you choose the best quality, so that a small portion satisfies you. And do note that some cakes and pies are lower in carbs than others: They contain less flour, less sugar and more fiber.

Food Item (Amount)	Carb (g)	Fiber (g)	Net Carbs (g)	Protein (g)	Fat (g)	Cals
Brownies						
Brownie mix, Atkins (2" square)	7.0	4.0	3.0	4.0	0.5	45
Pillsbury (1)	23.2	0.0	23.2	1.3	1.8	114
Sara Lee Brownie Bites (1)	12.0	1.0	11.0	1.0	4.0	90
Cake						
Angelfood, from mix (1/12 cake)	29.2	0.1	29.0	3.0	0.2	128
Cheesecake (1/12 cake)	20.4	0.3	20.1	4.4	18.0	257
CHEESECAKE, ATKINS						
Cappuccino (3 oz slice)	3.0	0.0	3.0	6.0	26.0	240
Chocolate Swirl (3-oz slice)	3.0	0.0	3.0	6.0	24.0	250
Raspberry Swirl (3-oz slice)	3.0	0.0	3.0	6.0	24.0	250
Strawberry Swirl (3-oz slice)	3.0	0.0	3.0	6.0	24.0	250
Vanilla (3-oz slice)	3.0	0.0	3.0	6.0	24.0	250
Chocolate cheesecake, Mrs. Smith's (1/6 cake)	50.0	2.0	48.0	8.0	37.0	550
Chocolate pudding, from mix (1/12 cake)	34.2	1.5	32.7	3.5	14.3	270
Devil's food, from mix, Pillsbury (1/12 cake)	33.0	2.0	31.0	2.0	14.0	270
Entenmann's Chocolate Fudge Cake (1 slice)	47.0	2.0	45.0	3.0	14.0	310
Entenmann's Sour Cream Chip & Nut Loaf (1 slice)	28.0	0.5	27.5	3.0	14.0	240
Gingerbread, from mix (1/9 cake)	34.0	0.8	33.2	2.7	6.8	207
Pepperidge Farm 3-Layer Vanilla (1/8 cake)	35.0	1.0	34.0	2.0	11.0	250
Pound cake w/butter (1/12 cake)	13.8	0.1	13.7	1.6	5.6	110

Food Item (Amount)	Carb (g)	Fiber (g)	Net Carbs (g)	Protein (g)	Fat (g)	Cals
Sara Lee All Butter Pound (1/12 cake)	14.0	0.0	14.0	2.0	6.0	120
Sara Lee Toasted Almond Cheesecake Bites (1)	8.0	0.0	8.0	1.0	6.0	90
Sponge, 16 oz (1/12 cake)	23.2	0.2	23.0	2.1	1.0	110
White, from mix, Betty Crocker (1/12 cake)	34.0	0.0	34.0	2.0	10.0	230
Yellow, from mix, Duncan Hines (1/12 cake)	36.0	0.0	36.0	3.0	11.0	250
Pie						
Apple, 9", frozen (1/8 pie)	42.5	2.0	40.5	2.4	13.8	296
Apple, Mrs. Smith's (1/8 pie)	56.0	2.6	53.4	3.0	17.0	390
Banana cream, 9", from mix (1/8 pie)	29.1	0.6	28.5	3.1	11.9	231
Blueberry, 9", frozen (1/8 pie)	43.6	1.3	42.3	2.3	12.5	290
Cherry, 9", frozen (1/8 pie)	49.8	1.0	48.8	2.5	13.8	325
Chocolate cream, 9" (1/8 pie)	44.3	2.8	41.5	6.8	22.9	400
Coconut custard, 8" (1/6 pie)	31.4	1.9	29.5	6.1	13.7	270
Lemon meringue, 9", homemade (1/8 pie)	49.7	1.5	48.1	4.8	16.4	362
Peach, 9", homemade (1/8 pie)	55.4	2.0	53.5	3.2	16.3	375
Peach, Mrs. Smith's (1/8 pie)	53.0	1.9	51.1	4.0	16.0	365
Pecan, 9", homemade (1/8 pie)	63.7	6.1	57.6	6.0	27.1	503
Pumpkin, 9", homemade (1/8 pie)	40.9	4.2	36.7	7.0	14.4	316
Pumpkin, Banquet (1/5 pie)	40.0	3.0	37.0	4.0	8.0	250
Rhubarb, 9" (1/8 pie)	45.1	0.0	45.1	3.0	12.6	507
Strawberry Cream Tart (1)	33.4	1.4	32.0	2.5	15.8	281

Food Item (Amount)	Carb (g)	Fiber (g)	Net Carbs (g)	Protein (g)	Fat (g)	Cals
Pie Crust						
Pie crust, 9", frozen (⅛ pie)	7.9	0.2	7.8	0.7	5.3	82
Graham cracker crust, 9" (⅛ pie)	19.2	0.5	18.7	1.2	7.3	145

SNACKS, COOKIES AND CANDIES

Stick to controlled carb snacks and candies, such as Endulge™ bars, and you'll do fine. Otherwise, it would be best to avoid foods in this category.

Food Item (Amount)	Carb (g)	Fiber (g)	Net Carbs (g)	Protein (g)	Fat (g)	Cals
Atkins Advantage Bar, assorted flavors	18-22	7-10	2-3	19-21	8-13	220-250
Candy						
Almond Joy Candy Bar (1.72-oz bar)	28.6	2.4	26.2	2.1	13.1	229
Andes Mints (8)	22.0	1.0	21.0	2.0	13.0	200
Endulge Caramel Nut Chew (1)	17.0	<1.0	2.0	6.0	9.0	140
Atkins Endulge Bar (1)	5.0	3.0	2.0	1.0	12.0	150
Atkins Truffle (1)	4.0	1.0	3.0	1.0	4.0	47
Cadbury Caramello (1.6-oz bar)	28.5	0.7	27.8	2.8	9.8	213
Cadbury Dairy (10 blocks)	24.0	1.0	23.0	3.0	12.0	220
Cadbury Fruit and Nut (10 blocks)	25.0	1.0	24.0	3.0	10.0	200
Caramel Twix (2-oz bar)	37.4	0.6	36.8	2.6	13.9	284
Chunky (1.4-oz bar)	22.8	1.9	20.9	3.6	11.7	198
Crunch (1.4-oz bar))	26.1	1.0	25.0	2.4	10.5	209
Good & Plenty (33 pieces)	31.0	0.0	31.0	1.0	0.0	130
Gumdrops (10 pieces)	35.6	0.0	35.6	0.0	0.0	139
Hard candy, all flavors (4 pieces)	23.5	0.0	23.5	0.0	0.1	95
Kisses (8 pieces)	22.4	1.3	21.1	2.6	11.6	194
Jellybeans (10 pieces)	10.2	0.0	10.2	0.0	0.1	40
Kit Kat (1/2 oz)	26.9	0.8	26.1	3.0	10.7	216
M&M's Peanut (10 pieces)	12.1	0.7	11.4	1.9	5.3	103
M&M's Plain (20 pieces)	10.0	0.4	9.6	0.6	3.0	69
Milk Chocolate (1½-oz bar)	26.1	1.5	24.6	3.0	13.5	226
Milk Chocolate w/Almonds (1.4-oz bar)	21.8	2.5	19.3	3.7	14.1	216
Milky Way (2.1-oz bar)	43.0	1.0	42.0	2.7	9.7	254
Peppermint Patties (3)	33.0	0.0	33.0	1.0	3.0	160

Food Item (Amount)	Carb (g)	Fiber (g)	Net Carbs (g)	Protein (g)	Fat (g)	Cals
Raisinets (20 pieces)	14.2	1.0	13.2	0.9	3.2	82
Reese's Peanut Butter Cups (2)	25.0	1.0	24.0	5.0	14.0	250
Reese's Pieces (20 pieces)	9.8	0.5	9.4	2.2	3.4	79
Snickers (2-oz bar)	33.8	1.4	32.3	4.6	14.0	273
Starburst Fruit Chews (5 pieces)	21.1	0.0	21.1	0.1	2.1	99
3 Musketeers (2.1-oz bar)	46.1	1.0	45.1	1.9	7.7	250
Twizzlers (3 pieces)	31.0	0.0	31.0	1.0	0.5	130

Cookies

Food Item (Amount)	Carb (g)	Fiber (g)	Net Carbs (g)	Protein (g)	Fat (g)	Cals
Animal Crackers/Cookies (15)	13.9	0.2	13.7	1.3	2.6	84
ARCHWAY						
Chocolate Chip (2)	11.3	0.0	11.3	0.7	4.7	87
Iced Molasses (2)	39.0	0.6	38.4	2.1	7.2	228
Oatmeal (2)	33.4	1.5	32.0	3.0	7.5	212
BARBARA'S						
Old Fashioned Oatmeal Crisp (1)	10.0	1.0	9.0	1.0	2.5	60
Traditional Shortbread Crisp (1)	3.0	1.0	2.0	1.0	4.0	80
Chips Ahoy! (2)	14.0	0.7	13.3	1.3	5.3	107
Dlightful Meringue Cookies (1)	0.0	0.0	0.0	0.0	0.0	0
Droxies (2)	14.0	0.0	14.0	1.3	4.0	94
Famous Amos Oatmeal Raisin (2)	10.0	0.4	9.6	1.0	2.9	68
Fig Bar (2)	22.7	1.5	21.2	1.2	2.3	111
Fudge Shoppe Deluxe Graham Crackers (2)	12.1	0.5	11.5	0.9	4.5	91
Ginger Snaps (2)	11.0	0.3	10.8	0.5	1.3	60
HEALTH VALLEY						
Chocolate Chocolate Chip (1)	13.0	2.0	11.0	1.0	5.0	100

Food Item (Amount)	Carb (g)	Fiber (g)	Net Carbs (g)	Protein (g)	Fat (g)	Cals
Peanut Crunch Oatmeal (1)	14.0	1.0	13.0	2.0	4.0	100
Keebler Oatmeal (2)	15.9	0.7	15.2	1.4	4.7	111
Lorna Doone (2)	9.5	0.0	9.5	1.0	3.5	70
NEWMAN'S OWN						
Champion Chip (2)	10.0	0.5	9.5	1.0	4.0	80
Fig Newmans (2)	13.0	0.5	12.5	1.0	0.8	60
Newman O's (2)	20.0	1.0	19.0	2.0	4.5	130
Nilla Wafers (2)	6.0	0.1	5.9	0.3	1.3	35
Nutter Butter (2)	19.0	1.0	18.0	3.0	6.0	130
Oatmeal, 2", from mix (2)	20.9	1.2	19.7	2.4	6.2	148
OREO						
Double Stuff (2)	20.0	1.0	19.0	1.0	7.0	140
Sandwich (2)	15.3	0.7	14.7	1.3	4.7	107
PEPPERIDGE						
Farm Bordeaux (2)	10.0	0.3	9.8	0.5	2.5	65
Farm Chessmen (2)	12.0	0.3	11.7	1.3	3.3	80
Farm Milano (2)	14.0	0.3	13.7	1.3	6.7	120
Sandies Pecan Shortbread (2)	18.2	0.6	17.6	1.9	10.6	175
Shortbread (2)	10.3	0.3	10.0	1.0	3.9	80
Sugar wafer with crème filling (2)	4.9	0.0	4.9	0.3	1.7	36
Vienna Fingers (2)	21.0	0.0	21.0	1.0	6.0	150
Walker's Shortbread (1)	11.0	0.0	11.0	1.0	6.0	100
Snacks, Savory						
Ultra Racquet Chips (6	4.0	0.0	4.0	0.5	1.0	30
CHEESE SNACKS						
Cheetos Crunchy (21 pieces)	15.0	1.0	14.0	2.0	10.0	160
Cheetos Curls (20 pieces)	20.0	1.3	18.7	2.7	13.3	200

Food Item (Amount)	Carb (g)	Fiber (g)	Net Carbs (g)	Protein (g)	Fat (g)	Cals
Just the Cheese (1 oz)	1.0	0.0	1.0	10.1	0.0	162
Robert's American Gourmet Pirate's Booty (1 oz)	18.0	1.5	16.5	2.0	5.0	128
CORN CHIPS						
Barbecue (20 pieces)	20.2	1.9	18.4	2.5	11.8	188
Fritos Original 20 pieces)	9.4	0.6	8.8	1.3	6.3	100
Onion rings, dry snack (1 oz)	19.5	0.0	19.5	0.1	6.0	134
POPCORN						
Cracker Jacks (1/2 cup)	23.0	1.0	22.0	2.0	2.0	120
Newman's Own Microwave Popcorn (1 cup)	4.6	0.9	3.7	0.6	3.1	49
Orville Redenbacher HomeStyle (1 cup)	5.0	2.0	3.0	1.0	2.0	35
PopSecret (1 cup)	4.0	1.0	3.0	1.0	2.5	40
Pork Rinds (20)	0.0	0.0	0.0	12.3	6.3	109
POTATO CHIPS						
Baked KC Masterpiece BBQ (15 pieces)	30.0	2.7	27.3	2.7	4.1	164
Barbecue (20 pieces)	13.7	1.1	12.6	2.0	8.4	128
Cape Cod Yukon Gold (1 oz)	19.0	1.0	18.0	3.0	5.0	135
Lay's Baked (15 pieces)	31.4	2.7	28.6	2.7	2.1	150
Lay's Classic (20 pieces)	15.0	1.0	14.0	2.0	10.0	150
Pringles Original (14 pieces)	15.0	1.0	14.0	1.0	11.0	160
PRETZELS						
Rods (3 pieces)	22.0	1.0	21.0	3.0	1.0	110
Soft (1)	38.4	0.9	37.5	4.5	1.7	190
Sticks (45 pieces)	21.6	0.9	20.6	2.8	0.9	103
Twisted (5 pieces)	23.8	1.0	22.8	2.7	1.1	114
Soybeans, roasted (2 tbs)	7.2	3.8	3.4	7.6	5.5	101

Food Item (Amount)	Carb (g)	Fiber (g)	Net Carbs (g)	Protein (g)	Fat (g)	Cals
TORTILLA CHIPS						
Doritos 3D Cool Ranch (20 pieces)	13.3	0.7	12.6	1.5	4.4	104
Doritos Nacho Cheesier (20 pieces)	22.7	1.3	21.3	2.7	9.3	187
Newman's Own Yellow Corn (1 oz)	19.0	2.0	17.0	2.0	7.0	150
Tortilla chips (20 pieces)	22.6	2.3	20.3	2.5	9.4	180
Tostitos Baked (20 pieces)	36.9	3.1	33.8	3.1	1.5	169
VEGETABLE CHIPS AND SNACKS						
Atkins Cruncher Snack Chips						
Sour Cream & Onion (1 oz)	8.0	3.0	5.0	12.0	3.5	100
BBQ (1 oz)	9.0	3.0	6.0	13.0	3.0	90
Nacho (1 oz)	8.0	3.0	5.0	12.0	3.0	100
Traditional (1 oz)	8.0	4.0	4.0	13.0	3.0	100
GeniSoy Soy Crisps (25 pieces)	17.0	2.0	15.0	7.5	2.0	110
Good Health Veggie Crinkle Chips (1 oz)	18.0	1.0	17.0	1.0	8.0	140
Robert's American Gourmet Original Veggie Chips (1 oz)	19.0	2.0	17.0	6.0	5.0	130
Terra Chips (1 oz)	18.0	3.0	15.0	1.0	7.0	140
Terra Stix (1 oz)	16.0	3.0	13.0	1.0	9.0	150
Terra Taro Chips (1 oz)	19.0	4.0	15.0	1.0	6.0	140
Top Banana Plantain Chips (1 oz)	17.0	2.0	15.0	1.0	8.0	130

BAKING PRODUCTS

Refined flour is very high in carbohydrates, so stick to a combination of ground nuts, soy and other protein flours and specially designed products. Note that spices like cinnamon and nutmeg are relatively high in carbs. When purchasing extracts, especially vanilla, be sure to look for natural flavors.

Food Item (Amount)	Carb (g)	Fiber (g)	Net Carbs (g)	Protein (g)	Fat (g)	Cals
Atkins Bake Mix (1/4 cup)	6..0	3.0	3.0	18.0	2	110
Baking powder (1/2 tsp)	0.0	0.0	0.0	0.0	0.0	0
Baking soda (1/2 tsp)	0.0	0.0	0.0	0.0	0.0	0
Chocolate, baking, unsweetened (1 oz)	8.0	4.4	3.7	2.9	15.7	148
Chocolate chips, semisweet (2 tbs)	14.4	1.3	13.0	1.0	6.8	109
Chocolate chips, semisweet, mini (2 tbs)	13.7	1.3	12.4	0.9	6.5	104
Cinnamon, ground (1 tsp)	1.8	1.3	0.6	0.1	0.1	6
Cocoa powder, unsweetened (2 tbs)	5.8	3.6	2.3	2.1	1.5	25
Coconut, shredded (1/4 cup)	3.1	1.8	1.3	0.7	6.7	71
Coconut milk, canned (1/2 cup)	3.2	1.3	1.9	2.3	24.1	223
Cornmeal (2 tbs)	13.4	1.3	12.1	1.5	0.3	63
Flour, all purpose (1/4 cup)	23.9	0.8	23.0	3.2	0.3	114
Gelatin, unsweetened, (1 envelope)	0.0	0.0	0.0	6.0	0.0	23
Ghee (1 tsp)	0.0	0.0	0.0	0.0	4.3	37
Molasses (1 tbs)	14.1	0.0	14.1	0.0	0.0	55
Sugar, brown (1 tsp)	4.5	0.0	4.5	0.0	0.0	17
Sugar, white (1 tsp)	4.2	0.0	4.2	0.0	0.0	16
ThickenThin Not Starch (1 tsp)	2.3	2.3	0.0	0.0	0.0	7

Dining Out

When watching your carb intake, it's easier to choose wisely in American or regional restaurants where familiar dishes are served. Ethnic restaurants present more of a challenge because food combinations, typical dishes and often, ingredients, are different. (Of course, that's why we opt for ethnic cuisines in the first place!) The charts that follow will help you make smarter choices. We've given guidelines, rather than carb counts,because recipes and portion sizes vary greatly from restaurant to restaurant.

General Guidelines:

• Don't arrive at a restaurant starving—it makes the contents of the breadbasket irresistible. To blunt your appetite, eat a hard-boiled egg or a few slices of cheese before you go out. Or, if you're on the run, snack on an Atkins™ Advantage Bar.

• Many restaurants feature their menus on-line. If possible, visit the Web site ahead of time to see if there are appropriate options and decide what you will order.

• Ask your waiter or waitress to explain any menu listings you don't understand. And keep in mind that most restaurants will substitute a portion of vegetables for potatoes, rice or pasta upon request.

• Ask for sauces on the side so that you can decide whether and how much to consume.

• Start your meal with a soup or salad—it will help fill you up. Likewise, drink plenty of water before your meal.

• Don't torture yourself if you accidentally consume something that's been batter dipped or breaded. Remember, it's only one meal.

• As far as dessert goes, you have two choices if you are beyond the Induction phase: fruit with unsweetened whipped cream or a golf-ball-sized portion of a "regular dessert." Otherwise, skip dessert—until you get home and can indulge in a controlled carb treat.

In Chinese Restaurants

Choose...	Instead of...
Egg Drop Soup	Egg Rolls
Shrimp Sizzling Platter	Shrimp Fried Rice
Steamed Tofu (bean curd) with Vegetables	Any Chow Fun (wide noodle) dish
Stir-Fried Pork with Garlic Sauce	Sweet and Sour Pork
Beef with Chinese Mushrooms	Any Lo Mein (narrow noodle) dish
Steamed Whole Fish (Sea Bass)	Shrimp with Black Bean Sauce
Chicken with Walnuts	Chicken with Cashews
Sautéed Spinach with Garlic	Moo Shu Vegetables (with pancakes)

NOTE:

If you're on Induction, stick to dishes that are stir-fried, steamed or broiled, and ask for sauces to be served on the side. On Ongoing Weight Loss, choose one sauced dish and one simply prepared dish. By the time you are on Pre-Maintenance and Lifetime Maintenance—and if your metabolism allows it–you may enjoy a half-cup to one cup of brown rice with your meal.

In French Restaurants

Choose…	Instead of…
Frisée Salad with Lardons (thin strips of bacon) and Poached Egg	Alsatian Tart (bacon, onion and egg pie)
Coquilles St. Jacques (scallops in cream sauce with cheese)	Langoustine en Croûte (lobster in puff pastry)
Moules Marinière (mussels in white wine and herbs) or Bouillabaisse (fish stew)	Vichyssoise (cream of potato soup)
Coq au Vin (chicken in wine sauce)	Canard a l'Orange or aux Cerises (duck with orange sauce or cherry sauce)
Entrecôte or Tournedos Bordelaise (steak in reduced shallot and red wine sauce)	Croque Monsieur (egg-dipped fried ham and egg sandwich)
Veal Marengo (veal stew with tomatoes and mushrooms)	Veal Prince Orloff (veal roast stuffed with rice, onions and mushrooms)
Haricots Verts au Beurre (buttered young green beans)	Pommes Anna (upside-down potato cake)
Assorted cheese plate	Crepes Suzette (crepes with orange butter and orange liqueur, served flambéed)

NOTE:

Southern French cooking, as well as bistro food, generally offers a wider range of choices than classic French cuisine because the preparations are simpler. In classic French, opt for beurre blanc sauces instead of béchamel sauces, because the latter contain flour. And beware of *frites*. These are what we call French Fries, are practically irresistible and arrive in heaps next to steak entrees.

In Greek Restaurants

Choose...	Instead of...
Tsatziki (yogurt and cucumber dip)	Skordalia (potato and garlic dip)
Avgolemono (chicken soup with egg and lemon)	Spanakopita (spinach and cheese pie)
Taramosalata (fish roe dip)	Dolmades (rice stuffed grape leaves)
Beef or Lamb Souvlaki (marinated, then grilled)	Moussaka (fried eggplant layered with meat and white sauces)
Roast Leg of Lamb, Grilled Lamb Chops or Braised Lamb Shanks	Pastitsio (casserole layered with pasta, meat and white sauce)
Chicken Grilled with Lemon, Garlic and Oregano or Rosemary	Chicken Pilaf
Braised Pork Loin with Lemon and Fennel	Any potato dish
Grilled Prawns, Octopus or Swordfish	Fried Kalamari (squid)

NOTE:

Instead of using pita triangles for dipping into *tsatziki* or *taramosalata*, ask for raw veggies. A good dessert option in Greek restaurants is a cheese platter. Cheeses such as Kasseri, haloumi and mizithra offer a variety of textures and flavors.

In Italian Restaurants

Choose...	Instead of...
Insalata frutti di mare (seafood salad)	Fried Calamari
Mixed Grilled Vegetables or Sautéed Portabello Mushrooms	Fried, Breaded Mozzarella Sticks
Arugula and Fennel Salad with Shaved Parmesan Cheese	Prosciutto with Melon
Antipasto (assorted meats and cheeses), Marinated Peppers and Mushrooms, Clams	Baked Stuffed Clams (usually bread-crumb heavy)

In Italian Restaurants (*cont.*)

Choose...	Instead of...
Escarole or Stracciatella (broth and egg drop) soup	Fettuccine Alfredo
Roasted Red Snapper or Salmon; Grilled Calamari, Shrimp or Scampi	Linguine with Clam Sauce
Grilled Chicken Paillard (boneless breast, pounded thin) or Pork Loin	Any risotto (creamy rice dishes)
Veal or Chicken Piccata or Scaloppini (very thin veal or chicken filets with lemon and capers)	Veal, Chicken or Eggplant Parmesan

NOTE:

Instead of nibbling bread while you peruse the menu, eat a few olives instead. And do as the Italians do: Start your meal with a bowl of soup (see choices above); it will help fill you up. The carb grams in tomato sauces vary widely, and can be quite high, so use your judgment: If a dish is buried in sauce, gently push some to the side.

In Indian Restaurants

Choose...	Instead of...
Shahi Paneer (homemade cheese in creamy tomato sauce)	Vegetable Samosas (pastries)
Roasted Eggplant with Onions and Spices	Any Pakora (fritter)
Chicken Shorba Soup (made with garlic, ginger, cinnamon and spices)	Lentil or Mulligatawny Soup
Any Korma (meat in cream sauce)	Any Biryani (rice dish)
Any Tandoori (oven roasted)	Any Pilaf (rice dish)
Lamb or Chicken Curry	Any Dal (lentil or bean dish)
Any Lamb, Chicken or Shrimp Kebab	Lamb, Chicken or Shrimp Saag (cooked with spinach and spices)

NOTE:

To start your meal, request some spiced cooked vegetables or a cooked cheese dish such as the Shahi Paneer (see chart). Inquire about all the ingredients in a specific dish because Indian food combines so many that menus do not list them all. "Vindaloo" dishes, which are spicy curries, often contain potatoes. In some restaurants, rice and lentils are served a la carte, while in others they are plated along with the entrées, so be sure to ask.

In Japanese Restaurants

Choose...	Instead of...
Oshinko (pickled vegetables)	Okonomiyaki (pancake-pizza)
Steamed Broccoli or Mixed Vegetables (no sauce), or Grilled Eggplant	Gyoza (fried vegetable dumplings)
Sashimi (raw fish without rice)	Sushi (raw fish with rice)
Shabu Shabu (meat and vegetables in broth)	Tonkatsu (deep fried pork)
Broiled Sea Bass (or any broiled fish of the day), soy or ginger sauce only	Shrimp Tempura (batter fried shrimp)
Miso (soy bean paste) soup	Seafood Soba or Udon (noodle soups)
Negamaki (green onions wrapped in paper-thin slices of beef)	Beef Teriyaki

NOTE:

Seaweed salad is a pleasant and mild tasting accompaniment to Japanese food, so try it (even if the ingredient is initially off-putting). Teriyaki sauce is sweetened with either corn syrup or sugar, so opt for plain soy sauce instead. Sip plenty of anti-oxidant-rich green tea with your meal. Its subtle flavor is best savored on its own, without sugar substitute.

Fast Food

Keep in mind that much fast food is highly processed, loaded with carbohydrates and often prepared with trans fats (hydrogenated oils). But sometimes, eating in fast food restaurants is unavoidable when you're on the go or don't want to make your friends or co-workers feel uncomfortable with your commitment to eating the controlled carb way. The fact is, you may end up in burger joints or pizza places from time to time, and so when you're in such a place, you should know how to choose the most nutritionally sound meal options.

To make things easy for you, we've reviewed menus from the top 10 quick-service chains, assembled lists of popular items and put the best possible choices in boldface type. We've also listed menu items that are higher in carbohydrate, so that you can see the vast difference in carb count between high- and lower-carb options. In some cases, you can "remodel" a fast food meal to reduce its carb count. For example, eating a burger without its bun can strip 29 grams of carbs off the tally. Although space does not allow us to include the full array of fast food companies, armed with the information provided, you should be able to "guesstimate" items at other chains. You can also check out their Web sites.

The nutritional analyses in this chapter come from the Web sites for included chain restaurants. In some cases, when we've "remodeled" an item such as removing the bun from a sandwich, we've estimated carb counts—we've double starred those items.

Burger Chains

At a burger chain, go with the flow and have a beef patty sandwich. Yes, even a bacon cheeseburger! Just toss the bun and be sure to order the burger "your way." Mayonnaise and mustard are permissible but watch the ketchup, which is often full of sugar. Watch out, too, for special sauces, as sugar often lurks in them as well. Slices of tomato and lettuce garnish are fine. Steer clear of anything advertised as "low-fat" because this label often translates to high carb. Also, make sure you avoid chicken sandwiches if they're breaded and fried. Salads are usually a sensible choice (but go easy on fast food salad dressings—most contain sugar or high fructose corn syrup, so make sure you read labels on the packets).

Food Item (Amount)	Carb (g)	Fiber (g)	Net Carbs (g)	Protein (g)	Fat (g)	Cals
McDonald's						
www.mcdonalds.com						
Cheeseburger (1)	36.0	2.0	34.0	15.0	14.0	330
Big Mac® (1)	47.0	3.0	44.0	24.0	34.0	590
**Hamburger patty (1)	0.0	N/a	0.0	12.0	12.0	110
Chicken McGrill® Sandwich(1)	46.0	2.0	44.0	26.0	18.0	450
**Chicken Fillet (1)	4.0	N/a	4.0	21.0	4.5	35
McSalad Shaker® Salads						
Chef Salad (1)	5.0	2.0	3.0	17.0	8.0	150
Garden Salad (1)	4.0	2.0	2.0	7.0	6.0	100

**estimated carb counts

Food Item (Amount)	Carb (g)	Fiber (g)	Net Carbs (g)	Protein (g)	Fat (g)	Cals
Burger King						
www.bk.com						
Hamburger (1)	30.0	2.0	28.0	18.0	14.0	130
Hamburger patty (1)	0.0	0.0	0.0	11.0	10.0	140
Whopper® (1)	53.0	4.0	49.0	29.0	39.0	680
Whopper® Patty (1)	0.0	0.0	0.0	25.0	23.0	320
BK Broiler® Sandwich (1)	52.0	3..0	49.0	30.0	25.0	550
BK Broiler® chicken breast patty (1)	4.0	N/a	4.0	21.0	4.5	35
Wendy's®						
www.wendys.com						
Classic Single® with Everything (1)	37.0	3.0	34.0	25.0	19.0	410
¼ lb. Hamburger Patty (1)	0.0	0.0	0.0	19.0	14.0	200
2 oz. Hamburger Patty (1)	0.0	0.0	0.0	9.0	7.0	100
Chicken Fillet Sandwich (1)	46.0	2.0	44.0	27.0	16.0	430
Grilled Chicken Fillet (1)	1.0	0.0	1.0	19.0	3.5	110
Arby's®						
www.arbys.com						
Regular Roast Beef Sandwich (1)	34.0	2.0	32.0	21.0	16.0	350
**Regular Roast Beef Sandwich without bun (1)	1.0	0.0	1.0	16.0	13.5	175
Grilled Chicken Deluxe Sandwich (1)	37.0	2.0	35.0	29.0	22.0	450
**Grilled Chicken Deluxe Sandwich without bun (1)	4.0	N/a	4.0	21.0	4.5	35

Food Item (Amount)	Carb (g)	Fiber (g)	Net Carbs (g)	Protein (g)	Fat (g)	Cals
Turkey Club Salad (1)	9.0	3.0	6.0	33.0	21.0	350
Grilled Chicken Caesar Salad (1)	8.0	3.0	5.0	33.0	8.0	230
Dairy Queen®/Brazier®						
www.dairyqueen.com						
DQ Homestyle Cheeseburger (1)	29.0	2.0	27.0	20.0	17.0	340
**Cheeseburger Patty (1)	0.0	0.0	0.0	15.0	14.5	180
Grilled Chicken Sandwich (1)	30.0	3.0	27.0	24.0	10.0	310
**Grilled Chicken (1)	4.0	N/a	4.0	21.0	4.5	35

Pizza Chains

The bad news is you'll have to forgo the pizza. The good news, however, is that many major pizza chains serve chicken wings that are relatively low in carbs. Order the wings, visit the salad bar and you've got yourself a meal. Select acceptable vegetables as a salad base, then top with protein foods such as hard-boiled eggs, turkey or chicken. Avoid coleslaw, which may contain sugar, and pass up that pasta salad. Use oil and regular red- or white-wine vinegar instead of a prepared dressing; commercial dressings often contain sugar and even balsamic vinegar has a smidgeon of sugar in it.

Baked stuffed potatoes are an absolute no-no. If it's absolutely necessary to order a pizza, eat only the cheese and fixings and leave the crust. It's a messy solution, but you'll avoid the nutrient-deficient high-carb crust.

**estimated carb counts

Food Item (Amount)	Carb (g)	Fiber (g)	Net Carbs (g)	Protein (g)	Fat (g)	Cals
Pizza Hut®						
www.pizzahut.com						
Mild Buffalo Wings (5 pieces)	<1.0	0.0	<1.0	23.0	12.0	220
Hot Buffalo Wings (4 pieces)	4.0	1.0	3.0	22.0	12.0	210
Pepperoni Lover's® Pizza (1 slice)	27.0	2.0	25.0	11.0	11.0	250
Veggie Lover's® Pizza (1 slice)	29.0	2.0	27.0	9.0	8.0	220
Domino's®						
www.dominos.com						
Buffalo Wings, BBQ (1 avg. piece)	1.5	<1.0	1.5	5.5	2.5	51
**Buffalo Wings, hot (1 avg. piece)	0.5	<1.0	0.5	5.5	2.5	45
Classic Hand Tossed Pizza (1/4 of 12-inch medium pizza)	55.0	3.0	52.0	15.5	11.0	375
Crunchy Thin Crust (1/4 of 12-inch medium pizza)	31.0	2.0	29.0	12.0	12.0	273
Ultimate Deep Dish (1/4 of 12-inch medium pizza)	68.5	4.0	64.5	23.0	27.5	598

Tex-Mex Chains

Mexican-style fast-food restaurants are tough territory, because most items include flour tortillas, which are high in carbs. So go armed with a fork so you can eat the fillings and push the tortillas to the side! It's difficult to calculate exact carb count but you can be sure that eliminating the tortilla will reduce it considerably. Your best bet is a taco salad, without, of course, the shell.

Food Item (Amount)	Carb (g)	Fiber (g)	Net Carbs (g)	Protein (g)	Fat (g)	Cals
Taco Bell®						
www.tacobell.com						
Taco	18.0	3.0	15.0	9.0	12.0	210
**Taco, w/out tortilla (1)	5.0	3.0	2.0	6.0	9.0	120
Taco Salad (10)	69.0	16.0	53.0	30.0	52.0	850
Taco Salad, w/out shell (1)	31.0	15.0	16.0	24.0	22.0	400

Sandwich Chains

Chicken or tuna salad is always a good choice. In sub shops, bring on the turkey, roast beef and cheese; steer clear of salami, bologna and other meat products preserved with nitrates. Ask for your selection on a plate instead of on a roll, and you're all set. Some sandwich chains will even leave off the bread and add your sandwich fillings to a salad.

Food Item (Amount)	Carb (g)	Fiber (g)	Net Carbs (g)	Protein (g)	Fat (g)	Cals
Subway						
www.subway.com						
Tuna Salad (1)	10.0	3.0	7.0	9.0	10.0	165
Roast Beef Salad (1)	11.0	3.0	8.0	12.0	3.0	114
Turkey Breast Salad (1)	11.0	3.0	8.0	11.0	2.0	105
Veggie Delight® (1)	9.0	3.0	6.0	2.0	1.0	50

**estimated carb counts

Chicken Chains

Here the challenge is to avoid anything that is barbecued or breaded. Barbecue sauce is typically full of sugar, and some of it has probably seeped into the meat. The safest thing is to remove the skin. Dry-rubbed meats are fine, or look for roasted chicken and acceptable side dishes, such as salad. If there's a grilled-chicken fillet sandwich available, grab it! Discard the bun, and you've got a pretty good selection. Or, if necessary, scrape the breading off a fried chicken breast.

NOTE: At KFC, it's better to scrape the breading off an "Original Recipe" chicken breast than a "Hot & Spicy" one—the total carb count will be lower.

Food Item (Amount)	Carb (g)	Fiber (g)	Net Carbs (g)	Protein (g)	Fat (g)	Cals
KFC®						
www.kfc.com						
Original Recipe® Chicken Breast Sandwich (1)	16.0	1.0	15.0	29.0	24.0	400
Hot & Spicy Chicken Breast Sandwich (1)	23.0	1.0	22.0	38.0	29.0	505
Tender Roast® Sandwich w/out sauce (1)	23.0	1.0	22.0	31.0	5.0	270